pregnancy

Fitness
MIND · BODY · SPIRIT FOR WOMEN

pregnancy

Fitness

MIND·BODY·SPIRIT FOR WOMEN

The Editors of *Fitness* Magazine
with Ginny Graves

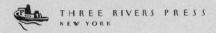
THREE RIVERS PRESS
NEW YORK

**Do not attempt an exercise or fitness
program unless and until you have had a thorough
examination and consultation with your physician. If you
experience any pain or discomfort during any of the exercises
recommended in this book, stop immediately and consult your physician.**

Copyright © 1999 by Roundtable Press, Inc., and Gruner & Jahr USA Publishing

Published by Three Rivers Press,
New York, New York.
Member of the Crown Publishing Group.

Random House, Inc. New York, Toronto, London, Sydney, Auckland
www.randomhouse.com

THREE RIVERS PRESS is a registered trademark and the Three Rivers
Press colophon is a trademark of Random House, Inc.

Printed in the United States of America

Design by Lauren Monchik

Library of Congress Cataloging-in-Publication Data

Pregnancy fitness / by the editors of *Fitness* magazine with Ginny Graves. — 1st pbk. ed.
Includes index.
1. Exercise for pregnant women.   2. Pregnant women—Health and hygiene.
3. Physical fitness for women.   I. Graves, Ginny.   II. *Fitness* (New York, N.Y.)
RG558.7 .P74   1999
618.2′4—dc21   98-50550

ISBN 0-609-80159-7
10 9 8 7 6

Credits

For Roundtable Press:
Directors: Julie Merberg, Marsha Melnick, Susan E. Meyer
Editors: Nancy Merberg, Meredith Wolf Schizer
Illustrator: Judy Francis

For *Fitness* Magazine:
Editor-in-chief: Sarah Mahoney
Fitness Director: Nicole Dorsey
Former Editor-in-chief: Sally Lee

Advisory Board:
Karen Andes, author of *A Woman's Book of Strength, A Woman's Book of Power,* and
    A Woman's Book of Balance, and coauthor of *Complete Fitness*
Joseph Apuzzio, M.D., Professor of Obstetrics and Gynecology at New Jersey
    Medical School and Director of Maternal/Fetal Medicine
Mark Fenton, Boston-based walking expert
Kathleen Little, Ph.D., Assistant Professor in the Department of Human Performance
    and Exercise Science at Youngstown State University in Youngstown, Ohio
James Pivarnik, Ph.D., Professor of Kinesiology and Osteopathic Surgical Specialties
    at Michigan State University and author of a number of studies on exercise dur-
    ing pregnancy
Bonnie Rote, R.N., B.S.N., Director of the Aerobic and Fitness Association of
    America's prenatal exercise education program
Cindy Schoenhair, Ph.D., Faculty in the Department of Health and Exercise
    Science at Paradise Valley Community College in Phoenix, Arizona
Mona Shangold, M.D., Director, Center for Sports Gynecology and Women's
    Health, Philadelphia, Pennsylvania
Julie Tupler, R.N., author of *Maternal Fitness*
Elizabeth M. Ward, M.S., R.D., spokesperson for the American Dietetic Association
    and nutrition counselor at Harvard Vanguard Medical Associates in Boston
Christine L. Wells, Ph.D., Professor Emeritus of Exercise Science at Arizona State
    University
Phillip Whitten, Ph.D., author of *The Complete Book of Swimming* and editor of
    Swimming World and *SWIM* magazines
Larry A. Wolfe, Ph.D., prenatal fitness expert and Director of the Clinical Exercise
    Physiology Lab at Queen's University in Ontario, Canada

The editors would also like to acknowledge the following institutions and indi-
    viduals for providing their time, research, and resource materials:
The American College of Obstetricians and Gynecologists; the American College
    of Sports Medicine; IDEA, The Health & Fitness Source; James Clapp III, M.D.,
    at MetroHealth Medical Center in Cleveland; and *Fit Pregnancy* magazine.

Contents

THE THIRD TRIMESTER

RECOVERING YOUR BODY

pregnancy

Fitness

MIND·BODY·SPIRIT FOR WOMEN

Introduction

No one can prepare you for what it feels like to be pregnant. Even if you've grilled all your friends and family about their experiences, even if you've actually read that stack of pregnancy books on your night-stand, even if you've been pregnant before, you probably *still* feel like you're in uncharted territory—that's because you are.

The truth is, no two women grow babies in exactly the same way. Some wrestle with morning (and afternoon and evening) sickness every day for several months. Others are ravenous from the moment those little cells start multiplying. Some love the way their expanding bellies look and feel. Others miss every inch of their old bodies, right down to their disappearing belly buttons.

We're here to tell you it's all normal—the highs, the lows, the anticipation, the tedium, the faith, the fear. It's just that your version of normal is as unique as your eye color or your taste in clothes. We're also here to provide you with a way to cope with the whole messy but miraculous experience—exercise. Even if you've never done anything more strenuous than carry a briefcase, you can benefit from doing a little extra physical activity now. And if you're one of those people who plan their weekends around workouts and race schedules, you can look forward to maintaining a high level of fitness throughout your pregnancy, even as you redirect that competitive energy toward the big event that lies roughly nine months down the road.

We're not recommending that you choose this particular year to train for a triathlon, or a 5K for that matter. We're not even suggesting that you work out every single day if you don't feel up to it. Our emphasis here is on moderate, do-as-much-as-you-can-and-then-go-put-your-feet-up exercise, which, when you think about it, is a good approach to take for just about everything during the tumultuous upcoming months.

"What's Exercise Got to Do with It?"

Good question. Why not just sit out the whole pregnancy, use the "delicate condition" clause in your mother-to-be contract, and take a hiatus from all but the most fundamental activities—brushing your teeth, for example—like Victorian women did?

Well, there are lots of reasons. For one thing, you may be nauseated for the first few months, and you will almost certainly feel dead-dog tired—*exercise can help.* For another, you'll be basting in hormones that can make you cry at the drop of a pencil. Again, *exercise can help.* Also, as your baby grows every day, your body is put under an increasing amount of physical strain, which can cause innumerable aches and ailments you've probably never even heard of till now. *Exercise can help.* And although you may not relish the thought, one day, not too very long from now, you're going to have to push something relatively large through a relatively small opening. *Exercise can help.* And someday, preferably before your baby graduates from high school, you're going to want to fit back into your favorite pair of jeans. *Exercise can help.*

In recent years, even doctors, who typically favor advice that's on the conservative side, have given the nod to exercise during pregnancy, based on the positive results of dozens of studies. The following are some relevant highlights:

• A study published in 1995 in the journal *Medicine and Science in Sports and Exercise* found that women who continued exercising three times a week for 30 minutes or more at a moderate intensity gained less weight overall and put on less body fat than women who quit exercising during their pregnancies.

• Researchers at the University of Iowa College of Medicine found that women who exercised three times a week for 20 minutes or more throughout the first two trimesters had significantly shorter—27 minutes versus 59 minutes—second, or "pushing," stages of labor than women who curtailed their physical activity during pregnancy.

• A study in the *American Journal of Obstetrics and Gynecology* looked at pregnant women who participated in a prenatal fitness program consisting of strengthening exercises and stationary cycling. The active women reported that exercise decreased the discomforts of pregnancy, relieved tension, and improved their self-image.

Sounds good, right? Still, a smattering of studies have come up with more sobering results—ones that make it clear that active pregnant women need to exercise common sense along with their quadriceps. Of at least eight studies looking for a link between exercise and preterm labor, just one found a small connection. That study, which followed pregnant women on active duty in the U.S. Army, found that those with the most physically demanding jobs—ones that required lifting 50 or more pounds at least 80 percent of the time—had a greater chance of delivering a preterm infant than women with lighter duties.

Meanwhile, in 1997, researchers at Indiana University found that strenuous exercise diminished the immune-boosting properties of nursing mothers' breast milk for up to 30 minutes after exercise. Their milk returned to normal about an hour after their workouts.

So, where does that leave *you*?

Fitness Q & A

To address some of the most pressing questions pregnant women have about exercise, and to clear up any lingering confusion you might be having about whether or not it's really worth it to get your fanny off the couch today, we went straight to some of the most eminent people in the field for advice.

1

Is exercise bad for my baby?

The answer is no, with a couple of important provisos. First, if you have certain pregnancy complications (see question #2 for details), you shouldn't exercise until you get clearance from your doctor. Second, if you're not physically fit to begin with, you'll need to go slowly. No matter what your prepregnancy fitness level, it's best to work at a moderate pace, because exercise that gets your heart rate above 150 beats per minute could cause your baby's heart rate to slow. Although this has never caused any actual damage so far as scientists can tell, why risk it? Meanwhile, you should limit the duration of your aerobic sessions to roughly 20 to 45 minutes, depending on your fitness and exertion levels. (In general, you can go longer if you work at a slower pace.) Prolonged aerobic exercise may cause the baby's temperature to rise, which could increase the risk of neural tube defects early in pregnancy or cause growth retardation later in pregnancy.

Is there any reason I shouldn't exercise?

Yes. The American College of Obstetricians and Gynecologists (ACOG) says that if you have any of the following conditions, you should take it easy during pregnancy:

• pregnancy-induced high blood pressure
• your water breaks before 36 weeks
• preterm labor during a previous pregnancy or your current one
• an incompetent cervix (one that opens prematurely under pressure from the growing uterus and fetus)
• persistent second- or third-trimester bleeding
• your baby isn't growing adequately
• you've had a miscarriage previously

In addition, women with certain other medical or obstetric conditions, including chronic high blood pressure, an active thyroid, or cardiac, vascular, or pulmonary disease should, in ACOG's words, "be evaluated carefully by a doctor in order to determine whether an exercise program is appropriate."

What are the best forms of aerobic exercise for pregnant women?

Walking is the ideal exercise, especially if you've been a couch potato up till now. Swimming is also great, because it's a non-weight-bearing sport and it improves your endurance and tones your muscles. Low-impact aerobics or yoga classes designed specifically for pregnant women are safe and have the added benefit of giving you a chance to compare strange, new symptoms with other mothers-to-be. Jogging is fine if you're used to it, but this isn't a good time to take it up, and cardiovascular exercise machines are a good option, provided you heed the advice about intensity and duration specified in question #1.

Are there any sports or activities I should specifically avoid?

Yes. Doctors say you should stay away from the following activities:

skydiving	contact sports	horseback riding
hang gliding	downhill skiing	field hockey
high diving	water-skiing	basketball
deep-sea diving	surfing	spelunking (cave exploring)
gymnastics	mountain biking	

Later in pregnancy, when your balance becomes iffy, you should probably also avoid softball, volleyball, in-line skating, ice-skating, tennis, racquetball, badminton, cross-country skiing, snowshoeing, step aerobics, and bowling.

 Can I lift weights?

Sure, if you're used to lifting weights. Just don't be macho about it. Lift only as much weight as you can manage fairly easily ten to twelve times. If you've never lifted before, stick with 2- to 5-pound handheld weights to build muscle strength.

 Is there anything I should do before I start exercising?

Check with your doctor. Tell her what type of exercise you'd like to do as well as your prepregnancy fitness routine to help her evaluate the safety and viability of your plan.

What This Book Can Do for You

We've created a trimester-by-trimester fitness program that will not only guide you safely through the whole nine months of pregnancy but also ease you back into fitness (and maybe even your old bathing suit) during that critical fourth trimester, when you find yourself learning to cope with a newborn *and* an extra 15 to 20 pounds.

Advice alert! The upcoming pages are chock-full of advice—a commodity you've undoubtedly found to be in abundant supply now that you're pregnant. If you're already on advice overload, here's our first suggestion: Pay attention only to news you can use. If you couldn't care less about hemorrhoids, say, or why some pregnant women develop sciatica, skim that section. That said, we think you'll find most of what we've included here profoundly interesting and absorbing—and useful.

A must-read: In the first section, we have a simple primer on the muscles that can make or break your pregnancy and delivery. Refer back to it any time you wonder why you really need to flex your pubococcygeus (PC) muscle, for example, or if you simply need to be reminded what the heck your PC muscle is.

With each new trimester, your body is going to throw you a curveball or two. From the fatigue and nausea of the first few months to the backaches and incontinence (no one ever said pregnancy was glamorous) that are common in the postpartum period, we address the physical changes of pregnancy, providing you with the most up-to-date medical advice in special how-to-cope sections.

You'll also find information on why your heart rate isn't the best gauge of exertion during pregnancy; how to assess your fitness level; how to get a safe, effective stretch; and how to buy a sports bra that fits your newly voluptuous self.

If you've already scanned parts of the book, you may have noticed a reference or two to our "Pregnant Brain" sections. You may have even wondered if we weren't a bit off track, including psychological stuff in an exercise book. We beg to differ, and here's why: While physical exercise bolsters your emotions as well as your abdominals, there may still be days when the idea of being someone's mother sounds about as appealing as having a Pap smear. The relaxation exercises we recommend here—meditation, progressive relaxation, and breath work—will help you rejuvenate your mental muscle on those days when your enthusiasm is a quart or two low *and* help you cope and stay focused once you're in labor.

At the end of each section, you'll find advice on aerobic exercise followed by your workout—a full spectrum of calisthenic-style toning and strengthening exercises that are geared specifically toward your most pressing needs and physical capabilities that trimester. For instance, in the first trimester workout, we pay special attention to strengthening your abs (for obvious reasons) as well as your leg and pelvic floor muscles, which will bear the brunt of the extra weight you'll be putting on in the upcoming months, while in the fourth trimester section we feature exercises you can do with your infant to tone and strengthen those stretched-out muscles. We also offer suggestions on how to modify each routine to suit your own fitness (or fatigue) level as well as recommendations and safety guidelines for stretching.

Whew! Feeling tired already? We wish we could tell you that simply reading about exercise would confer some health benefits. Unfortunately, turning pages doesn't offer much of a cardiovascular challenge. Until the day a book can do the work for you, let *Pregnancy Fitness* serve as the next best thing: a friendly, safe, and, we hope, enjoyable guide to getting the kind of exercise you need right now.

THE
first trimester

Your Changing Body

Your Fitness Profile

Nutrition for Two

Inner You

Cardiovascular Fitness

Getting Stronger

Enhancing Flexibility

1 Your Changing Body

Just when you're starting to get your mind around the fact that you really are pregnant, your body suddenly takes on a life of its own, changing at a rate that could make your head spin—that is, if you didn't already feel so dizzy and light-headed, thanks to the increased demands on your circulatory system. Sure, you knew your belly would eventually grow. But you may be astonished at the earlier, seemingly unnecessary havoc pregnancy wreaks on random body parts.

Instead of fretting over every new wrinkle, bump, and bulge, here's the thing you have to come to terms with: Pregnancy is a whole body phenomenon. Once you're pregnant, all of you is pregnant—your feet, your skin, yes, even your *hair*. If the idea of watching your old body go AWOL one cell at a time makes you feel like hyperventilating, console yourself with the knowledge that this parting of the ways doesn't have to be permanent, especially if you exercise and eat right over the course of the next nine months.

According to research conducted by James Clapp III, M.D., at MetroHealth Medical Center in Cleveland, women who continue to exercise throughout pregnancy gain less weight overall (although they gain a safe, healthy amount) and put on less body fat than their sedentary counterparts. In one of Dr. Clapp's studies, exercisers and nonexercisers gained similar amounts of weight through the fifteenth week, but between weeks 15 and 30, the exercisers gained an average of 1.25 pounds per week compared with 1.5 for the nonexercisers. Between weeks 30 and 37, the rate of weight gain slowed for both groups, but the exercisers still put on significantly less than the inactive women. In a separate study, Dr. Clapp found that exercising throughout pregnancy helps women recover more rapidly from labor and delivery and have improved VO2 max (a measure of fitness) at six months postpartum.

If you're worried about the safety of your little one at this early juncture, relax. Although most miscarriages typically occur during the first trimester, exercise doesn't seem to have anything to do with it. In fact, in one study, Dr. Clapp found that the miscarriage rate was actually lower—18 percent versus 25 percent—in runners and aerobic dancers than in women who stopped exercising during pregnancy.

That said, you have probably already discovered that these first few months are characterized by some rather *inconvenient* symptoms—ones that make the idea of working out sound about as appealing as dental work. (Look for our "How to Cope" boxes for specific advice on dealing with these fitness roadblocks.) Maybe you've been walloped by a fatigue so profound it makes blinking seem like an effort, or perhaps you're battling near-constant nausea, or you might simply feel emotionally off-kilter—all this, and your baby is still no larger than a lima bean!

Why all the upheaval already? Because your body started pumping pregnancy hormones into your system to spread the word that there's a baby on board *before* you even missed a period. Among other things, these early hormones cued your body to start building a placenta—a new organ, no less. This remarkable piece of equipment not only provides life support for your growing baby, supplying it with nutrients and oxygen, but also churns out pregnancy-enhancing hormones to keep your body in incubator mode (and your mind in la-la land) until your baby is big and strong enough to survive outside the womb. Meanwhile, that tiny creature that began as a handful of cells is growing into a real person, with arms, legs, tonsils, and toes. No wonder you're beat!

As if these sweeping changes weren't enough, they come part and parcel with lots of subtler alterations to your physical self, all of which need to be taken into account when you launch into this new era of pregnancy fitness.

Breast tenderness and swelling In the first few months of pregnancy, a surge of estrogen and progesterone signals your breasts to grow and produce *colostrum,* a pre-breast-milk concoction made up of water, protein, white blood cells, and protective antibodies that will provide early nourishment for your newborn (if you choose to breast-feed). The downside of nature's largesse: Your breasts may be tender and sensitive, a problem that usually disappears after the third or fourth month even though your breasts may continue to grow. Whether they're painful or not, your breasts need extra support now, even during minor bouts of exercise. If you don't already have one, or if the one you own is suddenly too small, now is the time to buy a supportive, well-fitting sports bra (see "How to Buy a Sports Bra" on page 64 for getting the right fit). Keep in mind, however, that you may have to invest in another one several months down the road. It's not unheard of for an A-cup wearer to blossom to a C- or even D-cup by the end of pregnancy.

Increased blood volume You've undoubtedly heard that you're eating for two (we'll tell you why that's not exactly accurate in chapter 3), but guess what? You're also pumping blood for two. That means your body actually has to produce more blood to meet the hefty demands of both you and your baby. In fact, by the end of your pregnancy, your blood volume will have increased by 30 to 50 percent, which simply means that your body is working harder than ever before. As a result, when you exercise you may tire more easily, even in these first few months when the baby is so small you don't actually look pregnant. You may also be prone to dizzy spells and light-headedness, because your circulatory system is expanding so quickly that your blood supply can have trouble keeping up, which can lead to low blood pressure. If you feel dizzy while exercising, stop and sit or lie down. If the dizziness continues, call your doctor.

Increased heart rate With all that extra blood being pumped throughout your body, your heart has to pick up the pace as well. In fact, your resting pulse rate may increase as much as 10 beats per minute during the first trimester, a change you'll feel even more acutely when you're exercising. Beware: Overexertion can cause an irregular or fast heartbeat, both of which are your cue to slow down gradually, allowing your heart rate to recover. If you feel dizzy, sit down.

Weight gain Prepare yourself. The scale may begin creeping up as early as the second month, especially if you breeze through the first trimester without any nausea or food aversions. For anyone who has worked long and hard to stay trim, these early pounds can be terrifying. Keep in mind that you're gaining weight for a good reason and that the alternative can have serious, adverse consequences. Women who are thin at the time they get pregnant and gain too little weight during pregnancy are more likely to deliver babies that are premature (their gestational age is less than 37 weeks) or of low birth weight (weighing less than 5.5 pounds); both conditions are more likely to lead to health problems that full-term, heavier infants are generally spared.

That doesn't mean you have carte blanche to consume an unlimited number of calories, however. Women who gain too much weight may face other difficulties, including gestational diabetes, high blood pressure, and even preeclampsia, a dangerous condition characterized by high blood pressure, fluid retention, and excess protein in the urine.

Some experts recommend that you put on 3 to 4 pounds during the first few months, but in reality, the rate of weight gain varies widely from woman to woman. You may gain no weight, or even lose some, during the first trimester, or you may put on 5 or 6 pounds. Trying too hard to tailor your progression to experts' suggestions can backfire by making you feel like a failure—the last thing you need right now. Here's a less rigid way to think about weight gain. If you were a normal weight when you got pregnant, you should try to adhere to a slow, steady increase, adding about a pound a week, starting in the second trimester, so that you put on between 25 and 35 pounds total. If you're carrying twins, your doctor may increase the range to 35 to 45 pounds.

With that in mind, check out this weight-gain advice from the National Academy of Sciences.

Prepregnancy Weight (in pounds)

Height	Underweight	Normal	Overweight	Obese
5′	<102	102–132	133–147	>148
5′2″	<107	107–141	142–157	>158
5′4″	<116	116–152	153–170	>171
5′6″	<123	123–161	162–180	>181
5′8″	<130	130–171	172–191	>192
5′10″	<138	138–181	182–202	>203
Pregnancy Weight Gain				
	28–40	25–35	15–25	15

Muscle Guide

Pregnancy, labor, and delivery are athletic events as surely as marathons and soccer matches are. They require muscle strength and endurance, commitment, and focus, all of which improve once you get into an exercise groove. That's why our workout routines have a decidedly athletic mind-set—we not only explain how to execute a particular move but also tell you which muscle(s) it targets, and why we've included it.

As a result, you're going to come across some fitness lingo as you flip through these pages. It's not meant to be intimidating. It's meant to be motivating. Our theory is that the more you know about your body and the "why's" and "how's" of exercise—why you need to strengthen your biceps, or how you'll benefit from strong pelvic floor muscles—the more likely you are to actually do it. We can't promise that if you strengthen a certain set of muscles or do X amount of cardio work your pregnancy or labor will be more comfortable, nor can we guarantee that you'll be spandex-ready by your six-week checkup. But we can assure you that the odds of having an easy time are on your side once you commit to a reasonable and safe fitness routine.

Don't know an ab from a lat? Think a trap is something you set for a mouse? Once you've read our muscle-by-muscle primer, you'll be able to *parlez* fitness like a real jock.

Abdominals (Abs) As your belly grows, your abdominal muscles are going to stretch, and like a rubber band, a muscle becomes weaker when it is stretched for a prolonged period of time. This is a concern for two critical reasons: (1) You really need strong abs to support the increasing weight of the baby and protect your vulnerable back, and (2) strong abs will give the muscles of your uterus some extra help when it comes time to push the baby out. Besides, unless you want to spend the rest of your life in pants with elastic waistbands, you really must learn to love (okay, tolerate) abdominal exercises, and the sooner the better.

Think of your abdominal muscles as a really elaborate girdle, running from the bottom of your breastbone down to your pubic bone and around to your ribs and hips. Your oblique muscles, which help you twist at the waist and bend from side to side, crisscross your midsection diagonally, with one set, the externals, extending from your rib cage to your pelvis, and the other set, the internals, running in the opposite direction from your pelvis to your ribcage.

Your transverse muscle, the innermost muscle of your abdomen, wraps straight around your midsection like a wide belt. It attaches at

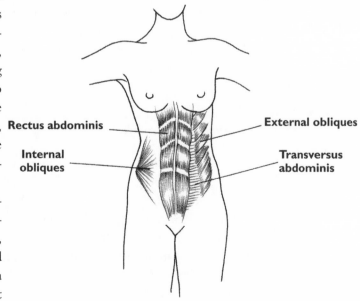

Rectus abdominis

Internal obliques

External obliques

Transversus abdominis

several points, including the top of your pelvis in the rear, the bottom of your lower six ribs, and the middle of your rectus abdominis, the parallel sheaths of abdominal muscle that run vertically up the middle of your belly.

As your pregnancy progresses, the vertical bands of the rectus abdominis may separate, resulting in a condition known as *diastasis recti*. It sounds more serious than it is, but it can be troublesome, leading to the backaches that plague so many women during and after pregnancy. In our upcoming exercise programs, we tell you how to check for a diastasis, how to modify your routine if you have one, and how to prevent it from becoming worse.

Pelvic floor muscles Think of these workhorse muscles as the hammock that cradles and supports your uterus, bladder, bowels, and other

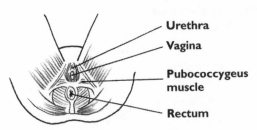

Urethra

Vagina

Pubococcygeus muscle

Rectum

pelvic organs. As your uterus grows, these muscles become overly stressed and start to sag, causing all sorts of potential problems, not the least of which is involuntarily peeing in your pants. Fortunately, it's fairly easy to strengthen the main muscle of the pelvic floor, the pubococcygeus, or PC, muscle, which forms a figure eight around the openings to the urethra, vagina, and rectum.

Not only does a strong PC muscle help you keep things like urine and all your internal baggage *in,* it will also help you push your baby *out.* Here's why: A strong muscle actually stretches more easily than a weak one, so when it comes time for your baby's head to make its appearance, and your muscles are being stretched in ways you couldn't imagine, you want your PC to be as supple (read: strong) as possible.

To find your PC muscle, pretend you're in the middle of urinating and just heard the final boarding call for your airline flight. The muscle you squeeze to stop the flow of urine is your PC muscle. In the routines we've created, you'll find a variety of pelvic floor exercises that will help you strengthen your PC muscle and, alternately, learn to relax it.

Back muscles With the exception of longshoremen and UPS drivers, most people don't spend much time thinking about their back muscles. During pregnancy, however, you end up carrying around 25 or so extra pounds without using your arms. Now *that's* hard labor. Not surprisingly, this extra load places an enormous amount of strain on your back, especially once your abdominal muscles start falling down on the job. To the rescue: strong back muscles.

The erector spinae are muscles that run the entire length of your spine, helping you stand up after you bend over to tie your shoe or, later on, when you lift your baby out of her crib or pick up his binky for the umpteenth time. They are also the muscles that can help counteract that oh-so-attractive pregnancy slouch—head jutted forward, shoulders rounded, lower back arched (more on this in the second trimester section)—that will set in once your baby is big enough to exert a gravitational pull on your body.

The other muscles that will aid in this task of keeping you upright while all the forces in the universe seem to be pulling you forward and down are the ones located primarily in your mid and upper back: the latissimus dorsi (lats), your largest back muscle, running from below your shoulders to your lower back; the trapezius (traps), a diamond-shaped muscle that drapes across your shoulders, neck, and center of your back; and the rhomboids, a small, rectangular group of muscles in the middle of your back.

Arm and shoulder muscles Babies, helpless creatures that they are, need lots of carrying. Eight pounds isn't a lot of weight, but it can feel like 800 pounds after you've toted your fussy newborn back and forth across the living room floor for several hours. That's why our exercise section includes moves that target the triceps (tri's), located at the back of your upper arms; the biceps (bi's), located at the front of your upper arms; the deltoids (delts), which wrap around the top of your arms; and the pectorals (pecs), which lie in front of your shoulders and underneath your breasts. (Strong pecs can also help support your breasts, which, by the way, may need some extra help after nursing.)

Leg, butt, and hip muscles As you start adding weight around your midsection, guess what bears the brunt of the load? That's right, your lower body. The toll of this extra burden, together with pregnancy-induced changes in your circulatory system, may be manifest in charming ailments like varicose veins and swelling—both of which, fortunately, can be partially relieved by exercise.

Strong gluteus maximi, or butt muscles (glutes), will help you lift your growing self out of the La-Z-Boy (at the end of pregnancy it's not hard to imagine getting stuck there), while strong gluteus medius (outer thigh and hip muscles), which lie at your hips, will help protect your pelvis, which becomes increasingly susceptible to injury as pregnancy hormones loosen the ligaments that normally hold it stable. Meanwhile, strengthening the main muscles of your legs—the quadriceps (quads) at the front of each thigh, the hamstrings (hams) at the back of each thigh, and your shin and

How to Cope with Nausea

Morning sickness. At least 50 percent of moms-to-be are afflicted to some degree with this inappropriately named ailment. If you have it, you know that the nausea it causes doesn't discriminate between morning, noon, and night. It usually strikes anytime it feels like it—when you get a whiff of a pungent smell, or when you get a little too hungry, or even for no apparent reason at all. Needless to say, it can wreak havoc on even the best-planned exercise program.

Doctors don't know why some women suffer the ups and downs of morning sickness. Possible culprits range from low blood sugar to low blood sodium. One new theory holds that it's nature's way of protecting the fetus from potential toxins found in typical nauseating foods like bitter vegetables and some spices. In other words, if a food makes you sick, it's because it contains something that could harm your baby. But the most well-accepted explanation is that it's caused by the crazy proliferation of hormones swarming through your system once that teeny embryo decides to take up residence in your womb.

The good news: Several studies indicate that women who are nauseated during their pregnancies are less likely to suffer miscarriages or stillbirths than women who aren't. We know, that doesn't make it any easier to live with. The surest cure is time. In most women, morning sickness clears up by the second trimester. Until then, here are some suggestions to help you settle your stomach—and maybe even feel well enough to work out:

• **Sniff out the offending odors.** Different smells set off different women, but certain ones—notably, coffee, perfume, and cigarette smoke—are almost universally gag-worthy. Identify any and all troublemakers and ban them from your house until your nausea subsides.

• **Try the lemon cure.** For some women, inhaling the scent of fresh lemon immediately after smelling a nauseating odor can ward off the need to vomit. Carry a lemon in your purse, gym bag, or fanny pack so you always have this antidote at the ready.

• **Eat early and often.** Hunger can trigger an attack, so getting a little food in your stomach before it starts to gurgle can go a long way toward preventing an episode. To that end, have a snack, even if it's just a saltine cracker or two, before you get out of bed in the morning; keep a small supply of food at your bedside for quick midnight fixes; and replace your traditional three squares with six or even ten or more small meals. Since exercise is likely to make you hungry, eat a little bit right before and after every workout.

• **If you can keep it down, eat it.** Don't worry too much about nutrition at this stage of the game. If Fig Newtons and ginger ale are the only foods that sound appealing, go for it. You can get your diet back on track as soon as you can keep food in your stomach. In the meantime, take a prenatal vitamin to make sure you're getting enough of all the essential pregnancy nutrients like folic acid and iron.

• **Try a little pressure.** The Sea-Band is a wristband designed to ease the queasiness of motion sickness by exerting pressure on the underside of the wearer's wrist. It reportedly helps about 60 percent of nauseated pregnant women as well. It is available at most drugstores.

• **Drink, drink, drink.** One of the biggest dangers of morning sickness is dehydration, which is bad for both you and the baby. When you exercise regularly, dehydration is even more likely because you lose fluids through sweat. Even if you can't stomach any solid food, make sure you get a steady supply of fluids into your system—at least eight 8-ounce glasses a day.

• **Ease into exercise.** The good news is that, for some women, a walk in the fresh air is just the ticket to calm a recoiling stomach. Now for the bad: Too much movement all at once could backfire, making you even queasier than before. *Everyone's different.* Start off slowly and pay attention to how your body feels. Focus on deep, even breathing and try to concentrate on the way your muscles feel when they move. Don't push yourself. Stop before you get fatigued. And remember: If you feel perpetually sick, and you're eating so little you're actually losing weight, skip exercise until you start feeling better.

calf muscles—will help you avoid many of the common knee and ankle injuries that befall numerous pregnant women in later months, and instead keep your legs looking sexy while the rest of you starts looking, well, let's say "maternal."

Fitness Q & A

1   *I've never exercised before. Is it safe to start now?*

Yes, provided that you get an okay from your doctor, and you ease into it slowly. To build your aerobic capacity, begin with a program of easy walking, swimming, or stationary bicycling—5- or 10-minute sessions—and add to it gradually. Guidelines from the American College of Obstetricians and Gynecologists (ACOG) on exercise during pregnancy indicate that it's better to get regular exercise, at least three days a week, than to do short spurts of activity followed by long periods of inactivity, and also to begin with low-intensity, low-impact, or nonimpact activities like walking or swimming. (For specific advice on creating an aerobic program, see chapter 5, page 51.) Take care not to get too winded or overheated, and always stop before you feel exhausted. When you're doing our strength routines, stick with the number of repetitions you can do comfortably.

I'm signed up to run a 10K when I'm three months pregnant. Can I do it?

Yes, actually, but only if you run that distance regularly. If you're normally a three-miler, it's best to pass on the 10K. This isn't a good time to push your body beyond what it's accustomed to. Furthermore, even if you are a committed distance runner, you may have to make an attitude adjustment before the event. Although a number of athletes have continued to compete safely throughout their pregnancies, we recommend that you curb your competitive urges until after the baby is born. Run instead at a moderate pace, and resist the temptation to rate your performance by your prepregnancy standards. Remember: You're supporting two cardiovascular systems now, and it's natural for your body to fatigue more quickly. If you can't carry on a conversation while you run, slow down. Drink plenty of water before, during, and after the race. And stop if you feel hot, fatigued, or light-headed.

I have had a previous pregnancy that ended in miscarriage. Is it still okay for me to exercise?

Check with your doctor. Miscarriages are so common—it's believed that as many as 30 percent of pregnancies end in one—that it probably won't preclude you from exercising during this pregnancy. However, if you have a history of repeated miscarriages, or if you miscarried as a result of some physical problem like an incompetent cervix, your doctor may recommend abstaining from exercise to be on the safe side.

I'm slightly overweight and am anxious about the excess pounds I'm already starting to gain. Can I use exercise for weight loss?

Absolutely not. Although many women use exercise to lose or maintain their weight when they're not pregnant, that should not be the focus now. Instead, your pregnancy exercise goals should be to maintain muscle strength and flexibility, improve or maintain cardiovascular fitness, improve your posture, and maintain a healthy body image. The good news: A study conducted at the University of Miami found that pregnant women who exercised expressed a more positive attitude than a sedentary control group about their facial complexion, physical stamina, strength, energy level, body build, and overall health. As if that weren't enough, the exercisers also continued to have a positive attitude toward sex, while the inactive women reported more negative feelings about sexual activities.

Before I knew I was pregnant, I took several grueling aerobics classes. Do you think I harmed the baby?

It's very doubtful. One of the concerns some doctors have about exercise during pregnancy is overheating, as animal studies have shown that high maternal temperatures increase the risk of certain birth defects to the fetus, such as neural tube defects that affect brain and spinal cord development. There's never been any evidence, however, that an exercise-induced rise in maternal temperature can harm a fetus. In fact, Dr. Clapp's research has shown that a pregnant woman's body undergoes certain adaptations that make thermal damage to a fetus highly unlikely. For one thing, your body begins to sweat at a lower temperature when you're pregnant, and this "sweating set-point" continues to fall as your pregnancy progresses. As a result, the rise in body temperature associated with a typical 20-minute exercise session is 30 percent less in women in their first trimester than in nonpregnant women, and as much as 70 percent less in women in their last trimester. In addition, early in pregnancy, your body mass and the amount of blood flow directed to your skin both increase—two changes that improve your body's capacity to release heat.

 I have exercise-induced asthma. Is it safe to use my inhaler when I'm pregnant?

Yes. In fact, the overriding concern here is that you control your asthma, rather than worry about the minute amounts of asthma medication you absorb systemically. Most maternal/fetal medicine experts advise women to stick with whatever therapy works. The most common approach is to take a puff or two of a bronchodilator-type inhaler (like Albuterol or Proventil) 30 minutes before your workout. If your usual prescription doesn't seem to control your asthma now that you're pregnant, discuss the problem with your doctor.

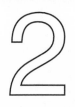# Your Fitness Profile

How fit are you, anyway? Wait! Before you toss off a quick answer, you really need to know what "fit" means. There are three components to fitness: aerobic capacity, strength, and flexibility. Think of them as the Holy Trinity. You need to be fairly competent in each element to be truly fit. That's not as easy as it sounds. Even a competitive athlete may have difficulty bending down and touching her toes, while a limber dancer is probably a poor bet in an arm-wrestling match.

Why measure your fitness level now? Several reasons. First, if you've never exercised before, you probably have no earthly idea what your body is capable of—how long you can walk before you start to get winded, at what point you break a sweat, how far you can go before your muscles start feeling like lead weights. Even if you exercise regularly, you may not have your finger on the pulse, so to speak, of your true fitness level, simply because you haven't had any good reason to pay attention to it. And even if you can recite your fitness stats right down to your resting heart rate, pregnancy deals your body so many changes that you might very well be playing with a whole new deck now.

By getting an objective sense of where you stand before you begin a workout routine, you can gauge your progression (or, as sometimes happens with pregnancy, your *regression)* along the way. Getting a read on your body's capabilities now will also help you make smart choices as you work to stay in shape throughout the upcoming months. You'll know when to push yourself a little harder, and, perhaps more importantly, when to call it quits. You'll have a better idea of which strength and stretching moves you can try, which you can modify, and which you should ignore.

First things first, however. Before you flex even one single muscle, you need to have a heart-to-heart with your doctor about your plans. If she isn't familiar with your full medical history already, let her know any health problems you've had, particularly any previous injuries or history of heart disease or high blood pressure, as well as any pesky ailments—a sketchy back, say, or weak ankles—that might have an impact on your fitness future.

Once your doctor gives you the okay, take these basic tests to gain some insights about your physical abilities. Although all of these moves have been shown to be safe during pregnancy, every woman's body responds to exercise in a slightly different way. At the first hint of dizziness, nausea, or an uncomfortable pulling in your abdomen or pelvis, *stop the exercise!*

One final word: We suggest that you buy a notebook in which to record your results. Trust us, it's virtually impossible to remember these stats while at the same time cramming as much baby-related information into your memory bank as possible, especially if you're a victim of the incredible shrinking brain syndrome (symptoms are forgetfulness and spaciness) so common during pregnancy. Besides, if you have a notebook, you can refer back to it and continue to add information to track your progress throughout your pregnancy and afterward—and there's nothing more motivating than positive results.

Testing Your Aerobic Capacity

What you'll need in order to gauge your heart's fitness: a watch with a second hand and a course that's one mile long. A local high school track works well, but if it's sweltering outside, opt for an indoor track or an early-morning outing. There's no sense getting overheated.

First, warm up by walking slowly for 5 to 10 minutes. Then, check your watch's second hand and walk your one-mile course as briskly as you can. If you weren't pregnant, we'd want you to push right on through any breathlessness or fatigue. But the rules are slightly different now, and it's important that you don't get too out of breath. If you feel yourself getting winded, do the "talk test"—have a little conversation with yourself or your baby. If you don't have enough breath to say, "I can't believe I'm talking to myself," you need to slow down.

When you finish walking the mile, check your watch again, and make a note of how long it took you. You can also check your heart rate (see "The Heart Rate Controversy," opposite). Keep walking slowly for 5 to 10 minutes after you finish the test. Stopping too quickly can cause blood to leave your head and pool in your legs—hence the term "light-headed."

Most people can cover a mile in 10 to 25 minutes. If you're at the high end of that range, or exceed it, your current aerobic capacity is fairly low. That means you'll have to pace your workouts accordingly, starting slowly and building your endurance gradually. The good news: If you continue to work out during pregnancy, you will probably see a big improvement over the course of the next few months. If you're toward the low end of that range, you're in good shape aerobically, and your goal should be to maintain that fitness level rather than improve on it.

The Heart Rate Controversy

Although most U.S. researchers feel that heart rate isn't an accurate gauge of exertion during pregnancy, since your heart is beating faster than normal, exercise physiologists in Canada believe it's an effective tool to monitor pregnant women's exertion levels. In fact, they have devised and tested the following heart rate ranges for various age groups. In numerous studies, these ranges have been shown to be safe. Researchers recommend you work at the lower end of the range if you're just beginning an exercise program and in late pregnancy.

Age	Heart Rate Range (beats per minute)
<20	140–155
20–29	135–150
30–39	130–145
≥40	125–140

Our feeling is that, while you shouldn't ever judge your exertion by heart rate alone, it's helpful to familiarize yourself with how a given heart rate feels. Then, you can use the heart rate ranges printed above as a guideline to the upper limits of what's considered safe.

To find your heart rate, take your pulse at your wrist directly below the base of your thumb, where you see a faint bluish line. That's your radial artery. After you've walked your one-mile course, as you're cooling down, rest the fingertips of your middle and index finger (don't use your thumb, because it has a pulse of its own) lightly on the radial artery of your opposite wrist, and count the beats for one minute. Heart rate is measured in beats per minute. Wait one minute, then take your pulse again. It went down, right? That's your recovery heart rate.

To find your resting heart rate, simply take your pulse when you're sitting around reading a book or watching TV or when you first roll out of bed in the morning. Again, during pregnancy you shouldn't rely solely on heart rate information, since your pulse is faster and will speed up even more as your pregnancy progresses, but these readings can serve as a rough guide to the range of what is normal for you now.

How to Cope with Fatigue

Even the most driven of women are felled by the near-universal torpor of early pregnancy. Why does such an extraordinary event leave you with so little energy to enjoy it?

Ironclad explanations are difficult to come by, but the most likely one is that your body is working hard to feather the nest in which your young one will lie for the next few months. Whether you know it or not, your uterus is being transformed into a five-star hotel complete with water bed, housekeeping, and room service so prompt it makes Marriott's look positively indolent. When you think about it, it's actually surprising you're able to do anything more strenuous than press the buttons on the remote control and the microwave.

Although there's no way to completely offset this energy-sapping activity, you can steal back small snatches of your old verve. We recommend a two-pronged approach that may seem paradoxical at first. But as you've probably already noticed, there's a lot about pregnancy that doesn't make much sense. First, try to conquer it with kindness. If you give in to your fatigue, it may just pay you back with a smidgen of vitality. Accept any and all offers of help, eat as nutritiously as you can, and spend every moment in one of two modes: sitting or sleeping.

Where does that leave exercise? We're so glad you asked. That's the second prong of attack. We recommend you try to sneak 15 to 30 minutes of light activity in every day. Ironically, fatigue can be amplified by too much inactivity, so your best defense might just be a good offense. Also, exercise prompts your body to release feel-good chemicals called endorphins, which can cut through pregnancy's purple haze, at least temporarily. Don't push yourself through a killer aerobics class or force yourself to go on an extended run. Just take a nice leisurely hike or a slow jog, even a stroll around the block, preferably in late afternoon when your biological clock has your body primed for a little physical activity. If you can exercise outside, do so to take advantage of the sun's energy-enhancing rays. Be sure to stop long before exhaustion overtakes you, and you may actually be able to ride that exercise high right through till night-time.

Feel like you're sinking farther into the fog? Hang in there as best you can, and take comfort in the thought that most women rediscover their internal energy reserves by the beginning of the second trimester.

Testing Your Strength

• **Upper body.** The bench-press test is just what it sounds like: a test involving a bench-press-style move. We've modified it here so you don't need to belong to a gym (with barbells and fancy machines) to get a sense of your upper-body strength. What you will need are handheld weights in the 2- to 5-pound range (they'll also come in handy if you want to increase the challenge of some of the moves in our workouts). If you don't have weights, use soup cans or bottled water instead.

Lie on your back with your knees bent, feet flat on the floor a comfortable distance from your rear end. **If you're in your second or third trimester, place several pillows behind your back, so your head and shoulders are higher than your abdomen, at about a 45-degree angle to the floor. If you feel dizzy even in this position, add another pillow.** Hold a soup can or weight no heavier than 5 pounds in each hand. Start with your hands at shoulder height, shoulder-width apart, elbows pointing out to the sides. The backs of your hands should be facing your shoulders. Extend your arms straight up toward the ceiling perpendicular to your body, until your elbows are only slightly bent. Lower the weights to the starting position. Repeat as many times as you can. CAUTION: Keep breathing as you do the move, exhaling when you push the weight up and inhaling as you lower it.

Record the number of times you can do the move. Remember, there is no right or wrong amount. If your arms tire after just three to five presses, you'll know that your upper body is an area that could use improvement. If you feel like you could keep on lifting, congratulations. Start doing our fitness routines, and you'll stay strong throughout your pregnancy—and be more than ready to meet the challenges of motherhood.

• **Middle body.** Check for a diastasis before you do this test, and, if you have one, skip it. (To determine whether you have a diastasis, see page 30.) In the crunch test, the point is to do as many crunches as you can. There's no time limit. In fact, you shouldn't try to do them too quickly and risk getting winded. What you'll need: an exercise mat or towel. Lie on your back with your knees bent and your feet flat on the floor, a comfortable distance from your rear end. Keep your arms at your sides with your hands flat on the mat. **If you're in your second or third trimester, place several pillows behind your back, so your head and shoulders are higher than your abdomen.**

To do your crunches, lift your head, neck, and shoulder blades upward, sliding the palms of your hands along the towel or mat 2 to 3 inches. As you lift, exhale and pull your abdominal muscles in toward your spine. Return to the starting position. (If you're propped up by pillows, focus on keeping the effort in your abdominals. It's easy to let your hip flexors, the muscles at the front of your hips, do the work from this position.) Continue doing this move until you feel the first twinge of fatigue in your abdominal muscles. Record your results.

A reasonably fit nonpregnant woman should be able to do at least fifteen to twenty-five crunches before collapsing in a heap. If you're way shy of either mark, it's important to work slowly to strengthen your abs. In any case, as you start doing the abdominal moves in the exercise routines in this book, use the results of this test as a guide to the number of crunches you can do comfortably.

• **Pelvic floor.** We explained to you how to find your PC muscle in the "Muscle Guide" (see page 16). Now's the time to see how strong it is. Sitting in a chair with your feet flat on the floor, your legs spread slightly, squeeze your PC muscle. Can you hold the contraction for 10 seconds? If so, your PC muscle is fairly strong. If, on the other hand, it starts to quiver and quake in less than 5 seconds, you've got some serious Kegels—exercises that strengthen your PC muscle—in your future. Record your results. This is one area in which you're bound to see remarkable improvements.

• **Lower body.** You're going to assess the strength of your thighs and glutes with the squat test. Hold a 5-pound weight (or a soup can) in each hand. Stand with your feet about hip-width apart, your arms hanging down at your sides. First, contract your PC muscle, then bend your knees until your thighs are parallel to the floor. If you're having trouble estimating how far to squat, put a chair behind you. When your butt touches the chair, you're down far enough. (We suggest you contract the PC muscle first to counteract the pressure squatting will put on your vulnerable vaginal area.) **If you're in your second or third trimester, do only a quarter squat: Bend your knees, sitting back on your heels, until your torso is a quarter of the way to the floor.** Return to the starting position and repeat. Keep your knees in line with your ankles. When you bend your knees, you should still be able to see your toes, or better yet, be able to lift your toes off the floor. Don't lock your knees when you stand up in between squats.

Stop when your muscles feel the first twinge of fatigue or when you're unable to maintain your form—if you lose your balance, if you start bending forward at the waist, or if your heels pop up off the floor. Record your results. This exercise is tough, so don't be disappointed if you can only do three or four. Just keep your results in mind as you begin the lower-body exercises in this book.

Testing Your Flexibility

• **Shoulders.** Hold a towel in your right hand. Point your right elbow toward the ceiling and reach your right hand down your back between your shoulder blades, so that the towel is dangling down your back. Now put your left arm behind you, with your left elbow pointing toward the floor. Reach your left hand up toward your right hand. Grab the towel as high up as you can. If you can reach all the way to your other hand, your shoulders are nice and flexible. If there's an inch or more of towel between your two hands, you are more likely to suffer from shoulder and neck pain, especially as pregnancy progresses, unless you make an effort to loosen the area. Now try the other side. Don't be surprised if one side is significantly more limber than the other. If you do our stretching routines regularly, you'll notice a big improvement on your tight side.

• **Upper back.** Lie on your back with your lower back touching the floor (or as close as you can come to it). Reach straight overhead with your arms, then drop them to the floor above you. If your arms touch the floor easily and your lower back stays in contact with the floor, your upper back is fairly flexible. If you can't touch the floor, or if your back arches when you try, you may be susceptible to upper back and shoulder pain—both of which are more likely now that your breasts are larger.

• **Lower back and hamstrings.** Sit on the floor with your legs together and reach your arms straight out toward your toes. Keep your spine as straight as possible (slumping is cheating!) and bend at the hips instead of the waist. If it feels like your belly is getting in the way, spread your legs slightly. If you can reach past your toes, you're superflexible and should take care not to overstretch as you do our stretching exercises. If you can touch or almost touch your toes, you're doing well. If you can't reach past the tops of your ankles, you may struggle with lower back pain.

• **Quadriceps.** Holding on to a wall or chair back with your left hand for support, kick your right foot up behind you and grasp it with your right hand. If your heel touches or nearly touches your rear, your quadriceps are nice and long. Switch hands and repeat the move with your left foot. If you can't come within a few inches of your rear, your quadriceps muscles are overly tight, a condition that can set you up for knee pain.

• **Calves.** Sit on the floor with your legs straight out in front of you, and flex your toes toward your body. If your toes actually point back toward you, your calves are fairly limber. If your toes point straight up or slightly away from you, your calves are tight, which makes ankle sprains more likely.

• **Achilles tendon and ankles.** Holding on to a bed frame, doorjamb, or some other immovable object, gently squat down on your haunches, so your butt is resting against your calves. Keep your weight on the outsides of your feet. If your heels pop up off the floor immediately, or you can stay in the position comfortably for only a few seconds, your Achilles and ankles are fairly inflexible, which also can make you susceptible to ankle injuries. WARNING: Don't stand straight up from this position, because it will place too much pressure on your knees. Instead, turn and place one knee on the floor, then push up, using your higher leg for support and your back foot for extra leverage.

How to Check for a Diastasis

A diastasis is a separation of the two halves of your vertical abdominal muscles, caused by the expansion of your uterus. To see if your muscle has separated, lie on your back with your knees bent and your feet a comfortable distance from your rear end. **If you're in your second or third trimester, place several pillows behind your back, so your head and shoulders are higher than your abdomen.** Place your fingertips an inch or two below your belly button, with your fingers pointing toward your feet. This is the point where the two sections of the abdominal recti muscles normally meet. Lift your head as high as you can. Exhale as you lift. If you feel a ridge more than two finger widths across running from your pubic bone to your belly button along the midsection of your abdomen, you have a diastasis. Still not sure? Press gently on the midsection. The area where your muscles are split apart will feel softer than the muscle tissue on either side. If you have one, you'll need to modify most of your abdominal moves by using a splint, a towel or long piece of cloth, to keep the two halves of your abdominal recti from moving farther apart.

3 Nutrition for Two

In general, growing a baby doesn't require extraordinary effort on your part. You don't need to think about building a placenta, say, or reminding those little cells to divide. Thanks to some blessed master plan, all of these tricky details are taken care of without your conscious help. But you *can* give your hardworking body a hand in this amazing effort. In fact, the single most important contribution you can make to your baby's (and your own body's) health and well-being is to consume a nutritionally balanced diet. Study after study has shown that good nutrition during pregnancy produces measurable health benefits for newborns.

Ideally, you started eating right or taking prenatal vitamins before you even got pregnant, but, let's face it, the world is not a perfect place. Don't sweat your prepregnancy habits too much, even if the only food pyramid you paid much attention to was the scoop of Häagen-Dazs balanced on top of a fudge brownie. That said, now would be a good time to rethink your diet priorities.

First, however, let's put the oft-quoted concept of eating for two into perspective. Although it's been misconstrued (probably by some ravenous pregnant women) to mean that you can, even *should,* consume twice the number of calories once you're pregnant, in reality it is nothing more than a catchy way of saying your baby eats what you eat. This can be a tough concept to get used to when you've spent a lifetime eating for one. Just keep reminding yourself that you're the Official Eater, not the *only* eater. Or maybe this image will help: You binge on Doritos, your baby binges on Doritos; you snack on carrots, your baby snacks on carrots. It's really that simple.

Want to know a trick to get you off to a good nutritious start during pregnancy? Keep a food diary for a week. Just write down everything you eat, even that Twinkie you snuck in when you thought no one was looking. Then, as you read this chapter, rate your diet against what the experts recommend. Are you getting enough of the important vitamins? Do you drink milk? If not, do you have another source of calcium? Do you consume enough calories, based on your activity level? And just how many servings of fruit and vegetables do you *really* eat, anyway? What you find may surprise you.

The Nutrients You Need During Pregnancy

During the first trimester, your baby does most of its *becoming,* for lack of a better word. It is transformed from a mass of rapidly dividing cells into a teeny person, complete with all the requisite pieces and parts of a human body. In the second trimester, the baby's internal organs continue to grow and develop slowly, and she starts to gradually put on weight. By the third trimester, the baby's main job is to gain weight (we should all be burdened by such a task!). Most babies go from about 3 pounds at the beginning of this trimester to around 7.5 pounds (the average newborn weight) by the end. What fuels all this growth? The calories in the food you eat, of course. But all calories aren't created equal. A baby needs certain types of food, namely ones that are jam-packed with nutrients, in order to thrive—which makes your job as Official Eater that much more important.

To start both you and your baby off on the right track, make sure you build up on these important pregnancy nutrients early on, and maintain a healthy consumption of them throughout pregnancy.

THE MOST IMPORTANT MINERALS

Iron Before you got pregnant, you were more likely to be deficient in iron than in any other nutrient, because you lost a sizable portion every month during menstruation. Now that you're no longer menstruating, you may think your iron needs have diminished. Not so. In fact, it's more important than ever to make sure you're getting an adequate amount, especially if you want to have the energy to continue exercising throughout pregnancy.

What makes iron such a nutritional necessity? This essential mineral is part of the hemoglobin that circulates in your red blood cells. Hemoglobin is a protein that carries oxygen to your baby and to the cells of your body, and oxygen provides both of you with the energy you need to function. In early pregnancy you don't need much more iron than normal. Since you're no longer menstruating, you actually have some extra stashed away. But because your blood volume doubles as pregnancy progresses, it doesn't take much to deplete your iron stores, especially in the later months when your baby starts stockpiling this important mineral in preparation for living outside the womb.

When you get too little iron, your blood isn't able to carry as much oxygen, which means there isn't as much energy available to fuel the work that's taking place inside your body. The result: iron-deficiency anemia, a condition that probably won't affect your baby but will affect you. In one of those interesting twists of fate, your body automatically gives your baby's iron needs precedence over yours. So while she/he is happy as a clam, doing baby aerobics in your uterus, you'll be lying on the couch wondering why you feel so doggone exhausted. If you think you have the symptoms of anemia—pallor, extreme fatigue, weakness, palpitations, and breathlessness—ask your doctor for a blood test.

Beginning in the second trimester, few pregnant women are able to get enough iron from food to meet the 30 milligrams nutritionists recommend you consume during pregnancy. (If you're anemic, your doctor may advise you to get 60 milligrams or more.) If you're a vegetarian, you may have a particularly hard time meeting your iron quotas. In fact, conventional wisdom now holds that most women should take an iron supplement starting in the second trimester. If your doctor advises you to supplement your diet with iron (usually ferrous iron), make sure you get the most out of it by taking it the right way. Here's how:
• Take it on an empty stomach with fruit juice that has lots of vitamin C or with water and a C supplement. Vitamin C boosts absorption of iron in your body.
• Don't take it with milk, tea, or coffee, all of which can interfere with iron absorption.
• Don't take it at the same time you take a calcium supplement, if your doctor has recommended that as well. Instead, take one with breakfast and the other with dinner.

A word of warning: For some women, iron supplements cause side effects such as nausea, constipation, and appetite loss—the last things you need when you're pregnant. If that happens to you, try taking it with meals, even though the iron may not be absorbed as well. If it still bothers you, talk to your doctor about a lower dosage, and take special care to include more iron-rich food in your everyday diet. (See the chart on page 36 for suggestions.)

Zinc This all-purpose mineral is important to digestion, metabolism, breathing, wound healing, and maintenance of skin and hair. (You may know it best as one of the latest-greatest remedies to shorten the course of the common cold.) During pregnancy, it plays an especially important role, helping in the formation of your baby's developing organs, bones, and nervous and circulatory systems. By eating a well-balanced diet, you will almost certainly get 15 milligrams of daily zinc, which is the amount doctors recommend. (See the chart on page 36 for good food sources of zinc.)

Calcium Thought your milk-and-cookies days were long gone? Think again. Pregnancy requires lots of calcium. It's important to start getting enough calcium early on, even though the baby's needs aren't as high when it's small, because researchers believe that during early pregnancy a woman's body has the unique ability to store additional amounts of this mineral for later use. There's a good reason your body adapts to pregnancy in that way. By late pregnancy, your growing baby starts guzzling calcium—as much as 300 milligrams a day.

If you don't get enough in your diet, guess who loses? Yep, you do. The baby will simply take calcium from your bones in a complex chain reaction designed by Mother Nature to ensure that the baby's needs are met. Losing too much calcium from your bones at this stage could set you up for osteoporosis later on.

Nutritionists recommend that you get *at least* 1,200 milligrams a day—up 200 milligrams from the prepregnancy recommendation. Fulfilling that extra requirement isn't difficult. Two hundred milligrams is just slightly more than half a cup of milk or yogurt, both of which provide about 150 milligrams. If you're lactose-intolerant (unable to digest milk products properly), look for lactose-reduced or lactose-free products, stock up on calcium-fortified juices and grains, and ask your doctor about taking a calcium supplement. Interestingly, new research indicates that taking a calcium supplement during pregnancy may decrease your chances of developing high blood pressure. (See the chart on page 36 for good food sources of calcium.)

THE MOST IMPORTANT VITAMINS

Folic acid Also known as folate, folic acid is an indispensable nutrient for the developing fetus, even as early as the first few weeks of pregnancy. In fact, it's the main reason so many doctors recommend you start taking prenatal vitamins when you're trying to conceive. Folic acid is necessary for cell division, which is the way the baby grows in its earliest days. Getting sufficient folic acid early on dramatically reduces the chance that your baby will have a neural tube defect like spina bifida, a condition in which the baby's spinal column doesn't completely close. In fact, it slashes the rate of all neural tube defects by about 50 to 70 percent, lowers the likelihood of cleft palate, and may reduce the risk of premature birth, one of the leading causes of illness and death in newborns. One study found that women who consumed less than 240 micrograms of folic acid were twice as likely to have a baby that was born prematurely.

During pregnancy, you need at least 400 micrograms of folic acid (the March of Dimes recommends 800 micrograms), double the amount you needed before pregnancy. Although it's possible to get the required amount through food alone, it's unlikely. That's why doctors recommend you take a supplement throughout pregnancy. If you're going to supplement with an all-purpose vitamin, use one specifically formulated for the prenatal period. Regular multivitamins might contain too little folate and too much of other nutrients (see the chart on page 36 for good sources of folate).

Vitamin B$_6$ You need this vitamin during pregnancy because it assists protein in building your baby's new cells. It's especially important for the development of fetal brain and nerve tissue. The recommended daily value during pregnancy is 2.2 milligrams, an amount you can get by eating a balanced diet. (See the chart on page 36 for good sources of B$_6$.)

Vitamin C Vitamin C is necessary to keep cells functioning normally; it is essential for the development of bones, teeth, and blood vessels; and it helps your body absorb iron from plant sources like green leafy vegetables. Still, you don't need to pop hundreds of milligrams to have a healthy pregnancy. In fact, you need only slightly more vitamin C now—70 milligrams versus 60—than before you got pregnant. (See the chart on page 36 for good sources of C.)

Vitamin B$_{12}$ Your need for vitamin B$_{12}$, which is essential for cell division and growth, goes up slightly during pregnancy. Doctors say you should get 2.2 micrograms now. Since it's found in foods from animal sources, such as milk, eggs, cheese, and meat, you'll need to find a reliable alternative source if you're a vegetarian. Some good options are a fortified breakfast cereal or a supplement. (See the chart on page 36 for good sources of B$_{12}$.)

Vitamin A A word of warning: Don't consume more than the recommended amount of 4,000 IU daily. Research suggests that consuming 10,000 IU may increase the risk of birth defects. Pay special attention to any nonprenatal supplements—some contain as much as 25,000 IU of vitamin A.

THE IMPORTANCE OF PROTEIN

All the cells in your developing baby's body are made up largely of protein. Likewise, this substance is essential in the construction of the placenta, and it is a main ingredient in the amniotic fluid the fetus floats in and swallows. As a result, your protein needs remain high throughout pregnancy. However, you don't need tons of *extra* protein now. The American Dietetic Association recommends eating 60 grams a day. That's just 10 grams more than the prepregnancy requirement. To put it in perspective, one 3-ounce patty of meat has 20 grams of protein, and an 8-ounce glass of milk has about 8 grams.

Even if you're a vegetarian, you shouldn't have a problem getting an adequate amount of protein if you consume a variety of legumes, grain products, vegetables, and fruits. To be safe, however, if you're not getting any animal sources of protein you should probably shoot for slightly more than 60 grams, since protein from nonanimal sources is more difficult for your body to use.

Important Pregnancy Nutrients

Nutrient	Pregnancy Needs	Food Sources
Iron	30 milligrams	Lean red meats, poultry, fish, whole grains, green leafy vegetables, dried fruits like figs and raisins
Zinc	15 milligrams	Lean meats, shrimp, oysters (*only* cooked ones), whole grains, yogurt
Calcium	1,200 milligrams	Skim milk, cottage cheese, yogurt, hard cheese, sardines, shrimp, dark green leafy vegetables, almonds, sesame seeds, tofu
Folic acid	400 micrograms	Dark green leafy vegetables, oranges, dried beans and peas, cashews, peanuts, asparagus, avocados, pineapple juice, eggs, lima beans
B_6	2.2 milligrams	Eggs, whole grains, lean meats, nuts, dried beans and peas, bananas, avocados, corn, oatmeal, yams
C	70 milligrams	Citrus fruits, green peppers, strawberries, tomatoes, Brussels sprouts, melons, mangoes, broccoli, papayas, baked potatoes, kiwis
B_{12}	2.2 micrograms	Lean meats, fish, crabmeat, cottage cheese, hard cheese, eggs
Protein	60 grams	Lean meats, poultry, fish, dairy products, eggs, grains, nuts and seeds, tofu and other soy products, dried beans and peas, lentils

Prenatal Vitamins: To Pop or Not to Pop

In essence, your body requires more of nearly every essential nutrient as it works overtime to support all the critical activity in your womb. As a result, the idea of popping a pill containing everything you need sounds attractive. It's a hedge-your-bets kind of option that appeals to most expectant mothers' better instincts. But do you really need to take a pill to have a healthy baby?

Probably not, say nutritionists. But that's contingent on one important factor: that you eat carefully and well. Unfortunately, research has shown most pregnant women typically get too little of a number of important nutrients, including vitamin B_6, folate, calcium, and iron. If, despite your best efforts, your diet leaves something to be desired, you definitely should take a prenatal vitamin. (Stick with true prenatal vitamins. Regular multivitamins often contain too little of certain substances like folate and too much of other substances, including vitamin A.)

Also, if you're prone to nausea during the first trimester, certain healthy foods, especially leafy greens like spinach, can be virtually impossible to choke down. If you're too nauseated to eat anything healthy, a prenatal vitamin is just the ticket to keep you nutritionally on track. Just don't let that little pill lull you into a false sense of security. It's all too easy to lose sight of your dietary priorities if you assume you're getting everything you need in a single gulp. And if you choose to go the real-food route, remember that you'll still need a folate and iron supplement, and probably calcium as well.

Calorie Requirements

A pregnant body burns through fuel faster than a nonpregnant one. In fact, it takes more than 85,000 extra calories over the course of the nine months to build a healthy baby. That sounds like a lot, but it's not. It works out to just 300 extra calories a day on top of what you normally consume. That's the equivalent of 2 ounces of turkey on two slices of whole grain bread topped with lettuce, tomato, and sprouts, or 1 ounce of cold cereal, a banana, and 1 cup of skim milk.

If you're exercising (and we hope you are), you'll need slightly more than that, and you'll need to make sure you eat regularly and often. Here's why: During exercise, pregnant women have a decrease in blood concentrations of glucose and insulin and a rise in free fatty acids. Normally, your body would respond to this condition, known as hypoglycemia, by producing more glucose. When you're pregnant, however, that natural response is blunted, especially during the second and third trimesters. As a result, serious hypoglycemia can occur if you don't eat something (preferably carbohydrates, which are quickly and easily converted to energy) immediately after a workout.

Symptoms of hypoglycemia include muscle weakness, lack of coordination, mental confusion, and excessive sweating. If you start feeling any of these symptoms during or following exercise, that's your cue to stop whatever you're doing and eat. By carrying a bagel, some raisins, or a banana with you at all times, you can easily fend off this potential problem.

How many more calories will you need if you continue to exercise during pregnancy? Well, that depends on how much you weigh, what activity you're doing, how long you do it, and how much effort you're putting into it—way too many variables to give any precise answer. The easiest way to tell if you need more calories is to pay attention to your appetite and the scale. If you're ravenous all the time, you probably need to eat more. Likewise, if you're not gaining weight at the recommended rate, your calorie consumption is too low.

For a more objective estimate of the number of calories you need, grab a pencil and a piece of paper. (Sorry, this requires a little math.) First, get a general idea of the number of calories you need normally by multiplying your prepregnancy weight by 12 if you're sedentary, 15 if you're moderately active, and 22 if you're very active. For example, a 120-pound woman would need 1,440 calories if she was sedentary, 1,800 if she was moderately active, and 2,640 if she was very active. (You can see how dramatically physical activity changes your caloric requirements!) Then add 300 (your daily pregnancy bonus calories) to your number.

Don't Eliminate Salt

You've probably made an effort to cut back on sodium in recent years, based on medical reports linking it to high blood pressure. And you may assume that during pregnancy you should avoid the salt shaker altogether, especially if you have some swelling. In this instance, you'd be wrong. You actually need more sodium during pregnancy (and lactation) than at any time of your life, partly to support the expanded blood volume that's circulating in your system. Animal studies have shown that when sodium is severely restricted during pregnancy, it inhibits the normal expansion of blood volume and, as a result, limits the baby's supply of nutrients.

If you're exercising and losing salt through sweat, you'll need to be especially aware of adequate sodium intake. Pregnant women should get at least 2,000 to 3,000 milligrams of sodium per day. Fortunately, that's not hard to do if you eat a normal diet. Studies show Americans typically consume at least 4,000 milligrams daily. To avoid eating too much, keep tabs on the salt content from unexpected sources like ketchup, packaged soups, and bacon.

For some rough estimates of what a number of typical activities are likely to cost caloriewise, see the following chart. Remember, you're looking at calories in a new way now. Whereas before you might have seen this chart as a weight-loss guide—the more calories you burn during exercise the more weight you lose—now you need to view it as a weight-*gain* guide. The idea is to replace at least as many calories as you lose through exercise.

The following figures are based on a person who weighs 150 pounds. If you weigh less, you'll burn fewer calories. If you weigh more, you'll burn more.

Exercise	Calories Burned per Half Hour
Swimming (slow to moderate pace)	270
Aerobics, high impact	240
Jogging	240
Tennis	240
Bicycling (slow to moderate pace)	200
Treadmill (moderate pace)	200
Stair climber (moderate pace)	200
Stationary bicycling (moderate pace)	170
Aerobics, low impact	170
Yoga	140
Walking (4 mph)	140
Water aerobics	140
Walking (3 mph)	120
Weight lifting (light to moderate)	100
Strolling	80

(Source: *Medicine and Science in Sports and Exercise* 25: 71, 1993.)

If you're gaining too much weight, don't panic—and *don't diet*. The American Dietetic Association recommends you follow these tips for cutting back safely:

• Substitute skim or low-fat milk, yogurt, and cheese for their higher-fat counterparts.

• Choose the leanest cuts of meat, poultry, and fish.

• Broil, bake, grill, or stir-fry foods instead of frying them.

How to Cope with Increased Urination

Have you memorized all the graffiti on the walls of your workplace bathroom? Does it feel like your bladder is roughly the size of a sesame seed? Welcome to the capricious world of pregnancy, where one minute you can feel perfectly in control, and the next as if your urges are controlling you.

Doctors attribute this lively symptom to a number of things, including the increased volume of fluids in your system, the improved efficiency of your kidneys (they're quicker to rid your body of waste now), and the increasing weight of your uterus, which is still sitting in your pelvis right next to—you guessed it—your bladder. Expect this annoyance to ease up as soon as your uterus ascends into your abdominal cavity, usually around the beginning of the second trimester. Until then, don't let a little urine stand between you and your fitness regimen.

• Drink a glass of water about 45 minutes before your workout. Then urinate right before you start. If you lean forward while you're going it will help your bladder empty completely.

• Some women find they get the dribbles in between trips to the bathroom. If that sounds familiar, wear a light pad in your underpants or tights to catch the drips.

• If you're going on a run or walk, plan your route around potential pit stops so you can relieve yourself along the way if you have to.

• Go when you feel the urge. Holding it can increase the chance of urinary tract infection (UTI), which can be hazardous during pregnancy. Increased urination, one of the hallmark symptoms of a UTI, is also a symptom of pregnancy, so you might not realize you need treatment. If you experience any of the following signs of a UTI, call your doctor: the constant urge to urinate accompanied by little urine; pain or burning during urination; blood in the urine; fever. Catching a bladder infection early is critical, because, if left untreated, it can progress to a more dangerous kidney infection.

• Don't cut down your fluid consumption to save yourself a few trips to the bathroom. You actually should be guzzling *extra* glasses now (doctors recommend eight to ten) to support the expanded fluid needs of both your body and your baby. Active women should aim for the high end of the recommended amount, since they're losing fluids through perspiration.

Your Fluid Intake

We've all heard the advice that we're supposed to drink eight glasses of water a day. And we've all nodded our heads and continued to drink our usual three or four—less in many cases. The truth is, it's tough to get that much water down in one day. Between running to the bathroom every half hour and endlessly refilling your glass, drinking that much just seems like a pain.

But now that you're pregnant, it's more important than ever that you try. In fact, if you exercise you should probably shoot for eight to ten glasses a day. Some experts say that for every half hour of exercise, you will need at least one glass of extra fluid to replace the amount that you lose through sweating. You will also need more in warm weather, when excessive perspiration is more likely.

Drinking plenty of fluids will not only help you avoid dehydration, a potentially dangerous condition during pregnancy, but also maintain your amniotic fluid and blood volume, aid digestion, ward off constipation, and reduce the likelihood of excessive swelling or urinary tract infections.

Following are some tips to help your daily fluid requirements go down a little easier.

• Remember that every glass doesn't have to be pure water. Dilute several with fruit juice and have a glass or two of skim milk as well. (Just watch your calorie count. An 8-ounce glass of skim milk has close to 90 calories.)

• Measure a gallon of water and pour it into a pitcher in the morning. Stash it in the fridge and keep sipping from it throughout the day.

• Don't drink more than two glasses at one time. It may make you feel bloated and could throw your body chemicals out of balance.

• Sip a glass throughout every meal and during your midday snacks.

• When you exercise, carry a container of water with you in a fanny pack or specially designed water pack.

• Put a full glass on your nightstand when you go to bed. Anytime you wake up, take a drink or two.

• Console yourself with the thought that you're spending half your time running to the bathroom now anyway. You might as well have something to show for your efforts.

BEVERAGES TO CONSUME WITH CAUTION—OR NOT AT ALL

Can't live without your morning cup of java? You probably don't have to. But if you're used to having a virtual caffeine IV going all day long, you'll have some adjustments to make now. Studies show that less than 300 milligrams of caffeine daily, or the equivalent of about two or three cups of coffee, is safe during pregnancy. Don't forget that many sodas and tea have caffeine as well.

Since caffeine acts as a diuretic, you can't count any caffeinated beverage in your daily eight. In fact, if you drink a cup or two of coffee or tea, you need to be extra vigilant about your intake of noncaffeinated fluids because you'll be losing more through urination.

Caffeine Content of Common Beverages

Brewed coffee*	230 milligrams
Decaffeinated coffee*	5 milligrams
Hot tea*	40–80 milligrams, depending on how long it steeps
Iced tea*	70 milligrams
Cola drinks*	12–40 milligrams, depending on the brand
Chocolate milk*	5 milligrams

*All 10 oz. servings

Herbal teas may seem like the virtuous choice if you're out to avoid caffeine entirely, but, surprisingly, some aren't safe during pregnancy. They may act as laxatives or cause uterine contractions or heart palpitations. Teas that are considered safe include chamomile, raspberry, and ginger.

You've probably also heard mixed messages about alcohol. While most books say to avoid it entirely, lots of doctors take a softer line and many pregnant women continue to drink in moderation. Who's right? The truth is, no one knows for sure. Most experts say you shouldn't drink even one drop of alcohol, not because they have proof that small amounts are harmful but because they *don't know* whether small amounts are harmful. In other words, the most cautious route is total abstinence. If you really miss a nice glass of wine now and then, wait until you're past your first trimester. Then limit your intake to half a glass.

Your Five Basic Food Groups

You know that ubiquitous triangle that's on everything from cereal boxes to soup cans? The Food Guide Pyramid is a great map to healthy eating for everyone but you. The American College of Obstetricians and Gynecologists recommends a modified version of those guidelines for moms-to-be. Here's a before-and-after look at the five food groups, plus suggestions for the number of servings needed to fulfill each requirement.

Daily Servings

	Regular Guidelines	Pregnancy Guidelines	Examples of One Serving
Grains	6–11	9–11	1 oz. cold cereal, ½ cup cooked pasta, ½ bagel, 1 graham cracker, ½ cup cooked rice, 2 rice cakes
Fruits	2–4	3–4	1 medium-size piece of fruit, ½ cup cooked, canned, or cut fruit, ¾ cup fruit juice
Vegetables	3–5	4–5	1 cup raw leafy vegetables, ½ cup cooked vegetables, ¾ cup vegetable juice
Meat, poultry, fish, dry beans, eggs, nuts	2–3	3	2 oz. meat, 1 egg, ½ cup cooked beans, ½ cup fish
Milk, yogurt, cheese	2–3	3	1 cup milk, 1 cup yogurt, 1.5 oz. hard cheese, ¼ cup cottage cheese
Fats, oils, sweets	use sparingly	use sparingly	

4 Inner You

One minute you're fuming at your husband for eating the last chocolate chip cookie, the next minute you're feeling all softhearted and puddley-eyed over a teeny pair of booties or a miniature stocking cap, and then you're mad at him all over again for failing to share your tender feelings. Welcome to the wonderful world of hormone overload, where mood swings are par for the course.

Your Pregnant Brain

If you're feeling a bit testy or sensitive these days, you're in good company. Rare is the pregnant woman who finds that her equilibrium *isn't* rocked, especially early on in these turbulent nine months. This is because your body is producing so many chemicals that suddenly erupt in early pregnancy. Although no one knows precisely which hormones are responsible for the unpredictable emotional landscape of pregnancy, it's likely to be a combination of the following usual suspects:

Progesterone Without this hormone, you wouldn't stay pregnant. Unfortunately, with it, you may wonder how you'll stay sane. Your body starts producing excess progesterone as early as the first week of pregnancy. Among other things, it signals your brain to cease menstruation and it decreases the contractability of your uterus. Researchers believe progesterone is also the chemical responsible for the erratic moodiness of PMS, promoting depression, crying, and mental confusion, so it's not surprising that it creates some emotional chaos during pregnancy, when levels are especially high. Other symptoms it's been linked to include fatigue and decreased memory capacity, hence the dippy forgetfulness you've probably been experiencing.

How to Cope with Gassiness and Bloating

Ah, the joys of pregnancy. As if it isn't enough to have your figure disappear, now you're wondering if your dignity might just go, too. Pregnancy hormones, particularly progesterone, are to blame for these unwelcome symptoms. One of the jobs of progesterone is to relax the uterus, which decreases the likelihood of uterine contractions until the baby is ready to be born. Unfortunately, it doesn't just act on the uterus; it affects all the smooth muscles in your body, including those of your stomach and intestines. As a result, your digestive system tends to get a bit sluggish.

Although these symptoms may make the idea of exercise less appealing, a workout may be just the thing to ease your pain and discomfort. A brisk, 20-minute walk can improve digestion, thus reducing gassiness and bloating. Other things that might help: Eat a number of small meals instead of three large ones, which tend to overtax your underperforming digestive system; try to eat slowly so you swallow less air; stay away from notorious gas-makers, including broccoli, some beans, cabbage, Brussels sprouts, greasy foods, high-fat foods, and carbonated beverages; don't hold gas in when it wants to get out or you'll make the situation even worse; and try rocking vigorously in a rocking chair, pushing off with your feet at the bottom of the chair's down-swing—for some reason this trick, discovered by doctors who treat patients recovering from abdominal surgery, seems to help gas pass from your system more easily. (And what better way to prepare for all those 3 A.M. rocking-chair feedings in your future?)

Prolactin Normally, amounts of this hormone fluctuate daily in about a forty-five-minute cycle in both men and women. But during pregnancy it continues to increase steadily so that by the time you give birth to the baby it will be ready to do its main job: maintain your body's production of breast milk. As for its behavioral effects, prolactin can cause mild depression and fatigue. If you choose to breast-feed after the baby is born, you'll feel the effects of prolactin even more keenly, as this hormone is a notorious libido-inhibitor.

Estrogen Breast tenderness and swelling are some of the first signs of pregnancy, and are the telltale trademarks of this quintessential female hormone. Estrogen increases rapidly throughout the first trimester and continues to rise throughout pregnancy. Although it is often thought of as an antidepressant, when estrogen levels fluctuate rapidly, it can cause anxiety and irritability. Sound familiar?

Human chorionic gonadotropin (hCG) The interplay between hCG and progesterone gives you all your signs of pregnancy. In fact, hCG is present at only one time in your life, and that's during pregnancy. As a result, it's the hormone most take-home pregnancy tests look for. It is also known as the placental hormone, because, as you might surmise, it is produced by the placenta. Its production steadily rises just after the fertilized egg begins to attach to your womb and then starts to decline around the twelfth week. Although hCG hasn't been implicated in any moodiness per se, its life span is suspiciously similar to that of morning sickness, leading some researchers to speculate it could be at least partially responsible for early-pregnancy nausea—and it's hard to be cheerful when you're spending half your time with your head in a toilet bowl.

Relaxation and Breathing Exercises

Can you believe the hormonal horde that's invaded your system? It's a wonder you're able to function at all! Although a mommy-to-be's moodiness poses no harm to the baby, it doesn't do much for your marriage or your motivation to exercise. Let's face it, when you're cranky you don't feel like doing much of anything.

That's why we'd like to offer you a few easy techniques to relax your body as well as your mind, and perhaps even smooth out some of the bumpier parts of the roller-coaster ride to come. These relaxation exercises can also help you deal with everyday stressors that you may be feeling ill-equipped to cope with, and sloughing off stress can be critical to the well-being of both you and your baby. Stress not only exacerbates the effects of those pregnancy hormones, but also may have an effect on your infant. Several studies have found a link between high stress and both premature delivery and low-birth-weight babies.

The bonus: By learning these relaxation techniques now, you'll handle pregnancy with more aplomb *and* you'll be better able to cope and stay focused during labor.

Meditation If you've never meditated before, here are a few facts you'll probably find reassuring right up front: It doesn't require a mantra, chanting, or a contorted pretzel pose. In fact, all it does require is 15 to 20 quiet, solitary minutes in which to . . . sit. What a concept!

In its simplest form, meditation involves concentrating on one thing—your breath, say, or a word such as "love," a candle flame, or even a simple movement, like you'd find in tai chi or yoga. This sort of focus works like a snake charmer's flute to lure your mind away from the barrage of thoughts, feelings, and sensory input that normally turn it into a three-ring circus. The goal is to keep yourself anchored in the present moment, not drifting off into fantasies of your baby or concerns about your lengthening to-do list.

Although meditation isn't a toll-free express lane to Nirvana, it can have some practical payoffs. Studies have shown it can reduce stress and anxiety, relieve the symptoms of PMS (which means it should work well during pregnancy, too), ease headaches, and help insomniacs get some restful shut-eye. And some of the less scientific benefits are easily as profound. For instance, meditation can help you know yourself a little better by giving you the opportunity to observe your thoughts, to watch your mind in action. In essence, it helps you develop an awareness of the present moment. Here are the simple steps to serenity:

• Find a comfortable spot to sit on the couch or on the floor, preferably somewhere out of reach of the phone and other distractions. You should try to keep your spine fairly straight (but not military stiff). A good way for beginners to do that is to sit with your back against a wall or the back of the couch. At the very least, prop some pillows behind your back. (This isn't supposed to be torture, and you don't want to get distracted by physical aches and pains.)

• Set a timer for just 5 minutes if this is your first time. The timer is helpful because you don't want to have to keep checking your watch to see how much time has passed. (As you continue meditating, work your way up to 15 to 20 minutes.)

• Place your hands on your belly, gently close your eyes, and breathe normally. (We recommend you start by using your breath as a focal point, because it's probably the easiest technique to get the hang of.) Focus on the feeling of air moving in through your nostrils and filling your belly, then moving out. Try to concentrate on your breath flowing in and out of your body. If you become aware that your thoughts are wandering, gently remind yourself to bring your mind back to your breath.

• Don't worry if you keep struggling with thoughts. That's perfectly normal. Just try to stay detached from their emotional content. A trick to try: "Watch" your thoughts as if they were a foreign film with no subtitles.

• When your timer goes off, slowly open your eyes and take a few deep breaths to reorient yourself.

Practice this technique every day for several weeks, and you should start feeling noticeably calmer and more in control.

Breath work Never thought much about the benefits of breathing? It's high time you did. Doctors have long known that breathing techniques, like Lamaze and the Bradley Method, can help women get through labor. But breathing correctly and well can be useful long before D-day as well.

You probably remember the basics of breathing from seventh grade science class: With each breath, you take in oxygen and release carbon dioxide. What you may not know is that poor breathing habits diminish the flow of these gases to and from your body, making it more difficult to cope with stressful situations. In fact, improper breathing can cause all sorts of problems, including depression, muscle tension, headaches, and fatigue, none of which you need right now.

People usually breathe in one of two ways: the wrong way or the right way. Chest breathing is the wrong way. It's shallow and usually irregular and rapid—the kind of breathing that takes over when you're anxious, worried, or stressed out. It doesn't allow a sufficient amount of air to reach your lungs, which means your blood doesn't get enough oxygen, your heart rate may increase, and your body's stress response clicks on.

Abdominal breathing is the right way. It's how your baby will breathe once it's born, and it's how you should try to breathe starting now. Here's how:
• First, tap into your breathing pattern by placing one hand on your abdomen and the other on your chest. Which hand rises the most when you inhale? If your chest hand rises, you're a chest breather. If your abdomen hand rises, you're already breathing fairly well, but you can use your breath to greater advantage by completing this exercise.
• Keeping your hand on your belly, practice breathing into your abdomen for several minutes until you get a sense of how it feels. Watch your hand rise and fall to make sure you're doing it correctly.
• Now, breathe deeply into your abdomen and pause slightly before you exhale.
• As you breathe out, count "one, two, three, four."
• Continue to count as you exhale for 5 or 10 minutes. Your breathing will gradually slow, your body will relax, and your mind will feel calm.

Do this exercise anytime you think about it, and check your breathing periodically throughout the day. If your breath has gotten stuck in your chest, focus on bringing it back to your belly. Over time you'll find this becomes more natural.

Self-hypnosis If you're like most people, you probably think of hypnosis as a conjurer's trick, on par with rabbits being pulled from hats. But the fact is, hypnosis is a totally natural state of mind, one that you probably experience dozens of times a day. A hypnotic trance is nothing more than a state of intense concentration with a reduction in peripheral awareness. If you've ever zoned out while driving or been so caught up in a movie that you felt disoriented leaving the theater, you've been in a hypnotic trance.

In hypnosis, you simply enter that state at will. Studies have shown that it can decrease the sensation of pain, including labor pain, alleviate stress and anxiety, and help people achieve goals like smoking cessation and weight loss. Although there are hundreds of self-hypnosis techniques, here's an easy one to try at home:

• First, think of a place that you've always found relaxing—the beach, maybe, or the woods, or even your bedroom as a child. Call it your "special place."

• Sitting comfortably in a chair, fix your eyes on a point slightly above your normal line of vision. Let your eyes lose focus and your peripheral vision narrow. Allow your eyes to close and your body to experience a feeling of drowsiness.

• Imagine you are in your special place. If you chose the beach, for instance, try to see the color of the sand and the water, smell the salty ocean, feel the breeze, hear the waves lapping against the shore. (This is not the time to worry about what you look like in a bathing suit.)

• Every time you practice this technique, try to make your special place a little more real by focusing on all the details.

If you practice regularly, your body will begin to relax quickly and easily every time you think of your special place. Once you're in labor, you can use this technique to stay calm and keep your muscles relaxed, which will decrease the sensation of pain.

Cardiovascular Fitness

We know that cardiovascular fitness can help you clear away some of that first-trimester fog and supply you with a regular hit of happiness, thanks to the endorphins released during heart-pounding activities. We know that labor, the wide-awake kind, is hard work (with or without drugs), but we also know that the more fit your heart is, the more energy and endurance you'll have for the event.

We even know why cardiovascular fitness helps during labor. A strong heart is better able to supply your hardworking muscles with freshly oxygenated blood, which keeps them primed for action. Scientific gobbledygook aside, perhaps the most important thing we know is this: Real women have testified to the fact that being fit helped them tolerate labor pain better and gave them the stamina to tough it out—the pain, the pushing, the whole enchilada.

That said, you need to know how to get fit (or stay fit, if you're already there). What's the best way to train your heart for the Great Labor Challenge? That's a multiple choice question, because, well, you have multiple choices. There is no single prescription, especially when it comes to cardiovascular exercise, and for good reason: Everyone's starting from a different place. If you've never exercised before, you can't play by the same rules as the woman who lives to sweat. And she won't follow exactly the same program as your average moderately active Jane.

The whole situation is complicated by the fact that the first trimester of pregnancy is a confusing time, sportswise. Aside from a certain voluptuousness, you probably don't look pregnant yet, and you're certainly not encumbered by the trademark belly that will soon make complete strangers smile knowingly at you on the street. Still, your body is different, and you definitely *feel* pregnant. And you probably feel something else, too: cautious. Chalk that emotion up to a newly budding maternal instinct, or maybe simple self-preservation. Either way, that little voice that's asking "What is my body capable of doing?" is one you should pay attention to. (Check out our "Sports You Can Do" chart on page 62 for details on activities that have received a thumbs-up from most experts.)

Thanks to years of studying pregnant women and how their bodies respond to exertion, scientists have come up with a few general principles that will help you answer that question for yourself.

The Seven Commandments of Pregnancy Fitness

1. Exercise regularly, not sporadically. The American College of Obstetricians and Gynecologists recommends you commit to at least three days of exercise a week. (We'd like you to shoot for five to six days a week, but only if you feel up to it. Let your energy level and your body direct your decisions.)

2. Monitor your intensity by using the Rate of Perceived Exertion scale (see page 63). Keep your intensity in the "somewhat hard" range or lower. Or, if you aren't used to exercising, an even safer method of gauging exertion is the talk test. If you can't grunt out a five-word greeting to your neighbor, slow down. Likewise, if you have enough breath to belt the National Anthem, you probably can push a little harder.

3. Stop exercising when you're fatigued (not exhausted).

4. Keep close tabs on how hot you are, especially during the first trimester, and stop if you feel overheated. You should also augment your body's natural heat dissipation system (better known as sweating), by drinking plenty of fluids before, during, and after exercise (approximately 16 oz. for each hour of exercise), wearing lightweight, loose-fitting clothing, and avoiding hot, humid environments.

5. Always stop exercising gradually by decreasing your intensity slowly. Slowing down gradually is less stressful to your heart and easier on your muscles. Stopping too suddenly, on the other hand, can cause blood to pool in your legs, making you light-headed.

6. Stick with activities you know. This isn't a good time to take up jai alai, for instance, or even step aerobics if you've never done it before.

7. Stop exercising and consult your doctor immediately if you experience any unusual symptoms. (See "When to Stop and Call Your Doctor," page 58.)

Beyond those basic safety-first guidelines, you need to remember the regular exercise fundamentals: Always warm up for at least 5 minutes before you begin to exercise, so you get the blood flowing to your muscles (which makes injuries less likely), and stretch thoroughly afterward. (Chapter 7 is chock-full of recommended stretches.) Once you've taken all those factors into account, you're limited only by how your body feels and a healthy dose of common sense.

So, are you ready to get sweaty? To help you get started, we've come up with specific advice targeted to two fitness levels and created sample fitness programs to go along with them. These aren't your only options. In fact, the playing field is virtually wide open. Remember, for the next few months the pressure is off to lose weight or squeeze into those size 6 jeans. And you're not out to break any land speed records or even set a personal best. In fact, whether you're a novice exerciser or a committed athlete, we'd like to encourage you to adopt a stop-and-smell-the-roses attitude toward exercise that will help you get back to what physical activity is really all about: having fun.

Guidelines for New Exercisers

Congratulations! Whether you've been overcome by a sudden health consciousness now that you're about to be a mother or you're simply panicking about weight gain because your Levi's are a tad snug, we're glad you've chosen this time to get active. Because your body isn't used to regular exertion, you're going to have to gear up slowly, however. (Sorry, there are no shortcuts to improved fitness, especially now that you're exercising for two.)

Since this is new territory for you, you're probably concerned about your physical capabilities, particularly if your last encounter with exercise was in high school gym class. Will you be gasping for air before you get to the end of the block? Will it take more time to lace up your sneakers than to break a sweat? Trust us, you'll be fine as long as you follow our pointers and take it slowly. Heart work doesn't have to be hard work—*if* you work smart.

In fact, the physical stuff is only half the battle. To launch a successful workout program during pregnancy it's easily as important to get in the right frame of mind. So, before we address the nitty-gritty physical aspects of exercise, let's get a few things straight on the mental front.

First, we want you to delete from your memory banks the most counterproductive phrase ever to enter the exercise lexicon: "no pain, no gain." If your muscles don't feel like wet noodles when you finish, it isn't a good workout, right? *Wrong.* In fact, there's nothing more certain to derail a new exercise regimen than overdoing it. Pushing your body past the point of mild discomfort is a bad idea for anyone, but it's a dangerous idea for pregnant women.

Along the same lines, temper your initial get-in-shape zeal with a healthy dose of discretion. In other words, start off slowly, and know when to quit. This won't be hard to do if your body starts rebelling at the first glimmer of sweat. But it'll be tougher if your first day of exercise feels surprisingly great, which often happens. Call it beginner's luck. Or maybe your system is so shocked to be moving, it doesn't know enough to feel bad. In any case, if your brain doesn't convince you to call it a day, you'll wake up the next morning with a new and profound appreciation of the word "arrrrgh."

Finally, jettison any notions of using exercise as a weight-loss device. Sure, physical activity can keep weight gain from getting out of hand, but you should never try to actually *shed* pounds during pregnancy.

In the following scenarios, we provide guidelines for how long and how often you should work out. If you tire before you reach our marks, stop. Don't feel guilty or bad, or worse yet, decide you're not cut out for physical activity and take up permanent residence on the couch. Think of it this way: If you're at the bottom of the fitness ladder, you have only one way to go. If you stick with our programs, you'll be climbing your way up quicker than you expected.

YOUR BEST OPTIONS

Walking There's no easier way to get moving than to walk. That's one of the reasons it's such a good choice for anyone who is new to exercise. You already know how to do it. (Although you may need some hints to help you do it the right way. See "Stride Right" on page 55 for pointers.) You don't need to join anything. You don't need to own any special equipment, except some comfortable shoes. You don't even need to do it all at once, since the latest research shows that you can reap health benefits from sneaking in 5 minutes here and 5 minutes there. To paraphrase Nike, you just need to do it.

Walking is considered weight-bearing exercise, because your legs support your body weight as you move. That's good because it strengthens your bones in addition to your heart and your muscles. But it can be harder on your joints, particularly your knees, than non-weight-bearing exercises like swimming or biking. If you feel pain anywhere, slow down or stop. And always take a postwalk physical inventory to tune into how the composite parts of your body are holding up. How do your knees feel? Are your feet pain-free? Is your back stiff? If any part of your body is balking, slow down or decrease your mileage, or do both. And be sure to stretch well after each workout. (See "How to Treat a Sore Muscle," page 74, for details on what to do if you injure yourself.)

Also, because of the dangers of overheating, particularly in the first trimester, take extra care not to get too winded or hot when you do this workout. If the weather is cool, layer your clothing so you can strip down as you start to sweat. Or join the legions of mall walkers (no stopping and shopping, please), who head indoors when the mercury drops below the comfort zone.

the program: To warm up, walk slowly for 5 minutes. Then walk at a brisk pace for 5 minutes. You should be able to carry on a conversation. If you can't, slow down. On the Rate of Perceived Exertion scale (see page 63), your effort should be a 5 or 6. To cool down, walk slowly for 5 minutes. Do this at least three days a week for up to six weeks. When you feel ready, increase your brisk walking segment to 10 minutes. Stay at that level for three to six weeks. Continue adding to your brisk segment in 5-minute increments until you reach 30 minutes total, including the warm-up and cool-down.

Stride Right

Thought you had learned everything there was to know about walking by the time you ditched your pacifier and Pampers? Think again. Good form is essential if you're going to make a walk a workout. Whether you're new to fitness walking or you've been around the block a few times, remember to walk this way:

• Walk tall, with your back straight, your head lifted, and your shoulders relaxed. When you're moving at an easy-to-moderate pace, lean forward slightly from the ankles, not from the waist. As your pace increases, lean forward from the hips and slightly from the ankles. Don't bend your back or lengthen your stride. Instead, take shorter, quicker steps.

• Think "strength from the center." Feel the power a strong abdomen lends your upper body by pulling your abs in slightly.

• With each step, strike the ground with your heel, then roll forward to the toe, pushing off at the end of your stride.

• When you push off, squeeze the glute of the back leg.

• Bend your arms at 90 degrees, and pump them in a controlled, forward motion, rather than waving them wildly side to side. Keep your elbows near your sides, and bring your arm back until your fist is at your pant seam, forward until your fist is chest high. Keep your hands out front with your fingers slightly cupped, so they are relaxed. They should brush lightly against your hips on the backswing. Use your arm movement as a natural metronome, letting it drive the rhythm of your feet.

• Be present in the moment. By focusing on your body—how your muscles feel, the flow of the movement—you can get an extra bit of effort out of your muscles, and, as a result, a better workout. The bonus: You'll be adopting a relaxing, meditative state of mind that will enhance your postexercise buzz.

Swimming Now is not a good time to try to learn to swim. But, assuming you know how to do the basic strokes—freestyle, or crawl, breaststroke, and backstroke—this *is* a great time to get your old Speedo out of mothballs and into the pool. Swimming is the quintessential non-weight-bearing exercise. You actually weigh 90 percent less when you're submerged than you do on land, making water the exercise environment of choice for people with knee or other joint injuries. (If you're not a swimmer, a water aerobics class or water walking program can be beneficial as well.)

Swimming is also a great choice during the first trimester of pregnancy, because it's virtually impossible to become overheated since most pools are kept between 78 and 82 degrees. (To be safe, check the temperature. Most pools have a thermometer in them. If yours doesn't, ask the lifeguard how hot it is.) If it's 85 degrees or higher, you stand a greater chance of overheating. Go slowly and make sure you keep close tabs on your own temperature. To do the workout below, you should be able to swim at least 500 yards. That's 20 lengths of a standard, 25-yard pool. Test yourself before you start, preferably at a pool that has a lifeguard in attendance, just in case.

the program: To warm up, always swim slowly for 5 to 10 minutes. For the first three workouts, swim 50 yards. Rest 1 to 3 minutes. Swim 25 yards with a kickboard. Rest 1 minute. Swim 50 yards. This workout should take you about 10 to 15 minutes. If it feels too easy, add distance. Just don't overdo it. For the next three workouts, swim 75 yards. Rest 1 to 3 minutes. Swim 50 yards with a kickboard. Rest 1 minute. Swim 75 yards. For the next three workouts, swim 100 yards. Rest 1 to 3 minutes. Swim 75 yards with a kickboard. Rest 1 minute. Swim 100 yards. As you feel ready, continue adding 25 yards to each section until your swim time totals 30 minutes.

Guidelines for Intermediate and Advanced Exercisers

Being fit going into pregnancy has enormous advantages. You're physically strong, you know what your body can and can't do, you probably have more energy than nonexercisers, and you've already carved out a niche for exercise in your life. Your biggest challenges now will be sticking with your program through the ups and downs of pregnancy (see "How to Stay Motivated," page 61) and knowing when to ratchet back your intensity. That's where the Rate of Perceived Exertion (RPE) scale comes in handy (see page 63).

Swimming Basics

For anyone who has achieved a level of skill beyond the basic doggy paddle, swimming is an excellent cardiovascular option throughout pregnancy. Still, there are some fundamentals that will ensure a safe, effective workout.

• Adopt the geriatric-style pool entry: the ladder. Diving may cause too much abdominal impact; jumping could force water into your vagina.

• Watch your back, especially during the later stages of pregnancy when doing the breaststroke or swimming with a kickboard could give you a backache, as they both cause your back to arch.

• Breathe easily. Freestyle will cause you to become winded most quickly, especially if you don't breathe correctly. Try to breathe through your mouth every two strokes. If you wait even four or five strokes, you'll tire too quickly. When you want to take a breath, roll your entire body to the side until your mouth and nose come out of the water (your arm stroke should actually create a little trough so you don't get a snoutful of pool). If you have a hard time catching your breath doing freestyle, slow down or try another stroke.

• Don't flail. Strive for nice, long strokes, especially when you do the crawl, because your arms provide about 80 percent of your propulsion—more than in any other stroke. Reach out as far as you can and pull all the way through the water, accelerating your hand speed as you go, until your hand brushes your thigh. Keep your elbows high. Your goal: to take fewer than twenty-five strokes in a 25-yard pool.

• Kick correctly. If you're doing the crawl, you want to kick up and down from your hips, not your knees. Don't kick too deeply or let your feet break the water's surface.

• Stop if you feel pelvic pain. Certain kicks, particularly the frog kick, may tweak your pelvis. If the frog kick is uncomfortable, try slowing down and keeping your legs closer together, or switch to another stroke.

• Skip the flip turn if you've never learned to do it correctly, or if it feels uncomfortable, which it may as your pregnancy progresses.

Since you're used to exercising, you know what "moderate to somewhat hard" exertion feels like—the intensity you should aim for during pregnancy. What you might find is that, whereas you could run 3 miles in 30 minutes if you were exercising somewhat hard before pregnancy, now you may cover only 2.5 miles in the same amount of time exercising at the same perceived intensity. Don't let that bother you. If you continue to exercise at that level during your pregnancy, you'll maintain most of your prepregnancy fitness throughout the upcoming months.

If you're a competitive athlete, the mental adjustment will be your biggest challenge. Remember the old nursery tale about the tortoise and the hare? Well, forget the hare. You're in Tortoise Land now. Incidentally, the upshot of that fable is the turtle wins, and that's exactly the bottom line in pregnancy. Slow and steady wins the race. It's time to downshift; put your body in an easy gear and punch in cruise control.

Sure, there are women who continue competing right up until the time they feel their first contraction. Our feeling is, unless Nike has you on retainer, you should put competing on hold now. You can still run in a 10K race if you want to, just don't *race* the race. Set aside your quest for personal bests until you're back on track after the baby is born.

Most doctors say you should limit your exercise to about 30 minutes. That's enough to reap cardiovascular benefits, it's fairly easy to squeeze into your schedule, and it won't leave you with so little energy you can't lift this book to read on. Even so, there are a number of experts who believe that time restrictions needn't be placed on pregnant exercisers, so long as you don't push yourself to the point of exhaustion. If you're used to exercising for 45 minutes or more, you can continue to do it. But if you don't recover within an hour or two, or you remain fatigued for the rest of the day, it's time to scale back.

No matter what your fitness level, you need to determine if your regular exercise routine is safe now. (See our "Sports You Can Do" chart for details, page 62.) If you've been doing something that's not on our list, check with your doctor before you make a final decision whether to continue or quit your program. If you decide it's time to switch to a new exercise routine, or if you simply want a change of pace, try our sample programs. They'll give you a good workout, and they're physician-approved.

When to Stop and Call Your Doctor

If you experience any of the following warning signs during exercise, your body is giving you a red flag. Stop exercising immediately and alert your medical caregiver.
• Vaginal bleeding
• Fluid leakage from your vagina
• Swelling of your hands, feet, or face
• Sudden, severe headache
• Dizziness or light-headedness
• Abdominal pain
• Severe pain in the pubic area
• Nausea or vomiting
• Uterine contractions
• Heart palpitations or extreme shortness of breath

YOUR BEST OPTIONS

Swimming For those of you who grew up splashing around in the pool, it may be hard to think of swimming as exercise instead of pure recreation. But the truth is, it provides most of the aerobic benefits of running, with many of the benefits of strength training thrown in for good measure, because you're actually pushing against the water as you move. Here's a handy rule of thumb to keep in mind if you're thinking about swimming for fitness: One mile of swimming is roughly equivalent to 4 miles of running. In other words, if you are able to run about 8 miles in an hour, you'd probably be able to swim 2, but the energy you would expend and the calories you would burn would be about the same.

Moreover, swimming works all the muscles of your body without straining your joints or connective tissue—an issue that becomes increasingly critical throughout your pregnancy.

The downside: Proper form is crucial to good performance. (See "Swimming Basics," page 57, for pointers.) If you can go from one side of the pool to the other all day long but you've never received professional instruction, now would be a good time to sign up for some basic swimming lessons.

the program: Swim 5 to 10 minutes at an easy pace to warm up. Then, swim 100 yards at a brisk pace. Since you can't use the talk test with your face in the water, you'll have to rely on the RPE. Keep your exertion in the moderate to somewhat hard range. Swim with a kickboard for 150 yards. Rest 2 minutes. (If you get too tired, rest after 75 yards, then continue.) Swim 200 yards at a brisk pace. Rest 2 minutes. Swim with a kickboard for 150 yards. Rest 2 minutes. Swim 100 yards at an easy pace.

Cross-Training Think of cross-training as a gussied-up word for a really simple concept. All it means is that, instead of sticking doggedly to one particular workout, you incorporate a variety of activities into your weekly program. It probably appeals to a certain personality more than others. If you are in good all-around shape and tend to tire of the same old routine, cross-training might be just for you. In any case, cross-training is a great choice during pregnancy because it works a variety of muscles, it gives your body a break from the same repetitive motions, *and* it busts the boredom factor, which helps keep your motivation high.

the program: The goal is to get in a 30-minute cardiovascular workout at least three days a week. The options include walking, jogging, biking, swimming, stair climbing, and low-impact aerobics class. Don't do the same exercise twice in a row. Go for a brisk walk on Monday, ride a stationary bike on Wednesday, and take a swim on Friday. If you're having a low-energy week, do the bare minimum: Walk for 15 minutes at lunchtime or after dinner at least three days. Always warm up by walking, biking, or swimming slowly for at least 5 minutes before you start exercising, and cool down with some stretches (see chapter 7 for suggestions).

Running/Walking If you're a committed runner, it's fine to continue your regular program (the jostling won't shake up your well-protected baby), as long as you keep your intensity moderate by using the talk test and the RPE and take care not to get too hot. Forgo hills if they push your intensity or temperature too high. Remember, you're running to maintain your fitness, not increase it. If it's cold out, dress warmly and shed clothes as you begin to sweat. Steer clear of ice and snow. Although a fall probably wouldn't harm the baby, it could hurt you, and you certainly don't want to have to go under anesthesia to repair an injury or take painkillers at this stage of the game.

Most doctors don't actually go so far as to *recommend* you run during pregnancy, because the impact can be tough on your joints, especially as you start to put on more pounds. A great substitute is the following running/

A Closer Look at Exercise Terminology

For those of you who have made it a point to avoid any and all fitness information for the past fifteen years or so, here's a thumbnail sketch of what most people already know about cardiovascular exercise: *Cardio* is shorthand for anything having to do with your heart; *vascular* has to do with the two networks of blood vessels that ferry blood around your system, transporting nutrients and oxygen to your baby as well as your own muscles and other tissues. Put the two together, as in "cardiovascular," and what you have is the circulatory system. What helps that important system function more efficiently is aerobic exercise.

Which brings us to the next vocabulary word: *aerobic,* a term coined by fitness expert Kenneth Cooper. It means, quite simply, "with air." When you place it before the word *exercise,* it means any repetitive activity that increases your heart rate and requires your muscles to use more oxygen. To get to that point, the exercise you choose needs to use your body's big muscles, especially the ones in your legs and butt.

If you're not in very good shape, or if you simply push yourself too hard, you won't be able to inhale oxygen fast enough to keep up with your muscles' need for it. At that point, your exercise switches from aerobic to anaerobic, which means you're working without air. That also means you wouldn't be able to pass the talk test, and that, of course, means you are working too hard. If you get to that wind-sucking point in your workouts, take a chill pill.

walking program, which eases you gently out of the fast lane. Think walking is sissy exercise? Once you've covered a couple of miles at a good clip—4 to 4.5 miles per hour—you'll probably change your tune. Start doing this program now, and by the next trimester you'll probably feel fine about retiring your running shoes until after the baby is born.

the program: Always walk for 5 minutes to warm up. Weeks 1 to 3: Run for 12 minutes. Walk for 3 minutes at a brisk pace. Run for 12 minutes. Walk for 3 minutes at a brisk pace. Walk for 5 minutes to cool down. Weeks 3 to 6: Run for 10 minutes. Walk for 5 minutes at a brisk pace. Run for 10 minutes. Walk for 5 minutes at a brisk pace. Walk for 5 minutes to cool down. Every few weeks, continue slashing 2 minutes off your running time and adding it to your walking time until you're walking at a brisk pace the entire 30 minutes.

How to Stay Motivated

Good intentions are like empty Ben & Jerry's cartons—the road to Weight Watchers is paved with them. Instead of ditching yours before you even hit the second trimester, heed this stick-with-it advice.

• **Set your sights low.** Fantasies about total rigorous commitment tend to remain fantasies, especially during the first trimester when you may not feel your best. Instead, make a *realistic* game plan—at least 15 minutes of cardiovascular work three days a week, for instance—even if ideally you're shooting for 30 minutes most days. That way, you're setting yourself up for success, not failure.

• **Make a pact.** Put your intentions in writing to reinforce your motivation. You can even make a chart and post it on the fridge so it's in your face every day. Place a big X on the days you achieve your goal(s). Keeping track of your commitment can be motivation in itself. But if you go for more tangible dividends . . .

• **Give yourself a big, fat (not fatty) reward.** Pavlov definitely had the right idea. There's nothing like a little positive reinforcement (a movie date with your guy, some new lipstick, a massage) to keep you coming back for more.

• **No self-flagellation!** If you slack off for a week, go easy on yourself. You are *not* a loser. You're pregnant, which means every once in a while you're allowed to wallow in complete and utter slothfulness.

Sports You Can Do—and How to Do Them

Far and away the best exercises you can do when you're pregnant are walking, swimming, and bicycling. They have a high fitness quotient and a low injury quotient, the precise formula to get you safely and healthfully through pregnancy. If those three don't blow your skirt up, however, it's time to move on to plan B. Following are the options included on that plan, along with conditions and caveats by trimester. Keep in mind that most of the warnings for the first and second trimesters apply during the third trimester as well.

Activity	1st Trimester	2nd Trimester	3rd Trimester
Aerobics	Can do high or low impact	Switch to low impact	Avoid quick moves
Aerobics, step	Watch temperature	Lower step to 6 inches	Lower step to 4 inches. Avoid jumps or explosive moves
Cross-country skiing	Not above 10,000 feet, because altitude can cause oxygen deprivation	Avoid hills and ice; stop if you feel pulling in your pelvis	Stick to easy trails
Golf	Not in midday heat	Quit if swinging hurts your back	Quit if swinging hurts your back
In-line skating	Wear protective gear; avoid hills	Stay on smooth surfaces	Stop if balance feels even slightly off
Rowing	Not in midday heat	Switch to machine	Decrease resistance; stop if back or pelvis feels achy
Running	Not in midday heat	Stay on smooth surfaces	Decrease intensity
Snow-shoeing	Dress in layers so you can strip down as you heat up	Take slow, controlled strides to keep your heart rate in check	Take ski poles along to help you balance
Soccer	Not in midday heat	Avoid slippery fields	Stop if balance feels even slightly off
Softball	Not in midday heat; don't slide	Don't play first base or catcher—positions that can involve contact	Stop if swinging is uncomfortable
Stair-climbing machine	Don't overheat	Stop if your lower back hurts	Stretch well to avoid leg cramps
Tennis	Not in midday heat	Scale back your intensity; don't reach for hard-to-get balls	Switch from singles to doubles; stop if balance feels even slightly off

Activity	1st Trimester	2nd Trimester	3rd Trimester
Volleyball	Not in midday heat	Don't dive for balls	Stop if balance feels even slightly off, or if jumping feels uncomfortable
Weight lifting	Don't strain or hold your breath	Don't do any moves that require lying on your back	Stick with light weights
Yoga	Don't strain or overstretch	Avoid back bends, moves on your belly, inverted poses, twists, and any moves that require lying on your back	See 2nd Trimester

Rate of Perceived Exertion (RPE)

0 No exertion at all

1 Very light exertion

2 Light exertion

3 Light exertion/ Light-to-moderate exertion

4 Light-to-moderate exertion

5 Moderate exertion

6 Somewhat hard exertion

7 Hard exertion

8 Very hard exertion

9 Very hard exertion/Extremely hard exertion

10 Extremely hard exertion

• **Mix it up.** Feeling bored? Go for a hike instead of your usual walk, or add one day of some new activity—swimming, stationary biking, a prenatal aerobics class. The bonus: Your body will benefit because every new activity uses slightly different muscles.

• **Team up,** preferably with a pregnant partner, who won't have her sights set on the Ironman competition, either. Working out with someone else is motivating not only because it's a lot more fun than going solo but also because it adds just enough of a guilt factor to get you out of the house on those days when you can think of a thousand things you'd rather do.

• **Go for inspiration,** not perspiration. Sure you'll tire of exercising if you do it within the same four walls day after day. But it doesn't have to be that way. Find things that inspire you—rousing vistas, rocking tunes, even something good to read if you're treading the treadmill or stair climber—whatever it takes to make your fitness more interesting.

How to Buy a Sports Bra

Bigger breasts need a bigger bra, especially when the bra in question is a sports bra, which tends to fit like a compression bandage anyway. Here's how to find one that fits:

• Small- and medium-breasted women (A- and B-cup) can go for a compression bra—a snap- or hook-free version that you pull over your head and that presses your breasts flat. If you wear a C- or D-cup, stick with an encapsulation-type bra, which has two cups like a traditional bra. The theory is, it's easier to minimize the bounce of two smaller masses than of one large one.

• When you try on the bra, give it the jump test. Do your breasts feel secure, or do they flop uncomfortably? Remember, when you work out, any jiggling you see in the dressing room is going to occur hundreds of times, and that can get decidedly uncomfortable. Stick with the most bounce-inhibiting version, even if it's not the most fashionable.

• Check the straps. Are they padded? Do they feel snug, but not tight? Are they adjustable? Look at the back. The wider the back, the more support the bra will give you.

• Make sure hooks and fasteners don't come in contact with your skin.

• The armholes should be large enough so the fabric doesn't chafe, but it shouldn't droop either. A good test: Swing both arms in circles, like a windmill. If the fabric droops, sags, or pinches, try another bra.

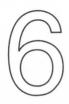 # Getting Stronger

Think of your muscles as your new best friends, or, better yet, as your new employers. You want to be really nice to them so that you get what you want out of them, namely support and power, in the coming months. You can do these exercises after you complete your aerobic work, or, if you can't spare an hour at a time, do your strength and aerobic work on alternate days. In any case, do the full routine at least three times a week if you have the energy, in order to keep your muscles strong. Every day try to do at least the basic curl-ups, Kegels, and plié or wall squat.

The following routine offers full-body strengthening and toning, but it emphasizes the muscles of your lower body, which need to be strong now to support the excess weight you're going to be carrying around shortly. (Don't you just love to be reminded?) For the floor work, it's helpful to have an exercise mat or at least a towel underneath you to provide some cushioning. We recommend you buy ankle and handheld weights in a variety of sizes, from 2 to 10 pounds. If you don't want to make that kind of investment, you can substitute water bottles or soup cans for real weights.

Even beginners should be able to do all these moves. If you're just starting out, however, stick with the minimum number of repetitions and sets, or do fewer if your muscles start to tire sooner. As you get stronger, you can add to your program. If you're an experienced exerciser, work at a somewhat harder level, but stop if anything feels uncomfortable.

REVERSE FLY

Muscles it targets: Traps, rhomboids, and lats.

Why do it: It strengthens the muscles in your upper back that help pull you out of the pregnancy slouch.

How to do it correctly: Fold a towel and place it over the top of the back of a kitchen chair. Stand about 2 feet behind the chair with your feet shoulder-width apart, your left foot about a foot in front of the right. Lean forward so your left forearm is resting on the towel and your forehead is resting on your arm. Bend your knees slightly and keep your spine straight. Holding a weight in your right hand so your palm is facing your right leg, allow your right arm to hang straight down from your shoulder toward the floor. Raise your right elbow up and out to the side by squeezing your shoulder blades together. When your right elbow is in line with your right shoulder, pause and slowly lower. Exhale as you lift; inhale as you lower the weight. Do 8 to 12 reps. Repeat using the left arm. Work your way up to three sets.

Things to bear in mind: Focus on squeezing the muscles in your back together during the movement. Keep your wrists straight throughout.

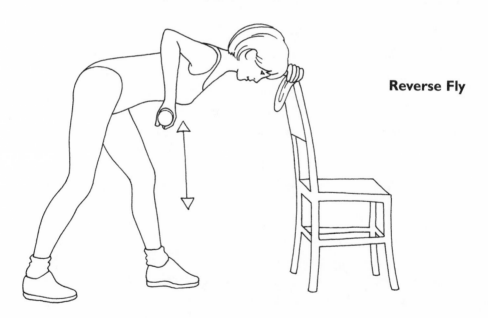

Reverse Fly

BICEPS CURL

Muscles it targets: Biceps.

Why do it: Biceps are muscles that assist your back muscles when you lift things, like a baby, or when you pull things—a suitcase through an airport, or a vacuum out of a closet.

How to do it correctly: Stand with your feet shoulder-width apart, your knees slightly bent, and your abs pulled in firmly. Hold your arms at your sides with your palms facing toward your thighs, a weight in each hand. Bending your arms at the elbow, raise both weights while rotating your palms toward your chest. Keep your elbows close to your waist. Exhale as you lift; inhale as you lower. Repeat 8 to 12 times. Work your way up to three sets.

Things to bear in mind: If you feel dizzy, sit in a chair to do this exercise. Don't hunch or slump your shoulders; don't rock your body or arch your lower back. Keep your wrists straight.

To make this move slightly harder: Use heavier weights. Squeeze your biceps at the top of each move.

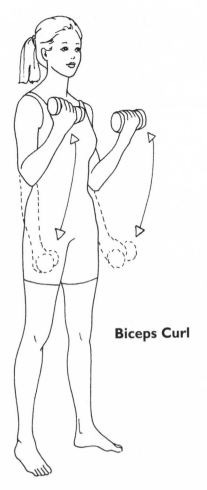

Biceps Curl

TRICEPS EXTENSION

Muscles it targets: Triceps.

Why do it: To ensure that the word *jiggle* doesn't apply to your arms.

How to do it correctly: Stand with your feet shoulder-width apart, your knees slightly bent, and your abs pulled in firmly. Holding a weight in your right hand, start with your right arm extended straight up overhead. Exhale as you lower the weight behind your head until it's even with your left ear. Keep your elbow pointed toward the ceiling. Inhale as you return your arm to the starting position. Do 8 to 12 reps. Repeat using the left arm. Work your way up to three sets.

Things to bear in mind: Keep your wrists straight so your triceps are lifting all the weight. Keep your upper arm stationary and don't lift the working shoulder.

To make this move slightly harder: Use heavier weights.

UPRIGHT ROW

Muscles it targets: Traps, delts, and lats.

Why do it: Strong shoulder and upper back muscles help you stand up straight and give the illusion of a smaller waist. (Why not enjoy it while you can?)

How to do it correctly: Stand with your feet shoulder-width apart, your knees slightly bent, and your abs pulled in firmly. Hold a weight in each hand at thigh level in front of you, the palms of your hands facing toward your body and the ends of the weights together. Take a breath, then exhale as you draw the weights upward, leading with your elbows until the weights are just below your chin, and your elbows are as high as your ears. Inhale as you lower the weights to the starting position. Repeat 8 to 12 times. Work your way up to three sets.

Things to bear in mind: If you feel dizzy, sit in a chair to do this exercise. Also, be careful not to arch your back, or to pull your shoulders out of alignment.

To make this move slightly harder: Use heavier weights. Lift and lower slowly to work the muscles thoroughly.

CALF RAISE

Muscles it targets: Calf muscles.

Why do it: Strong calf muscles will help support your additional weight in coming months, especially when you walk and run. Also, since women in later pregnancy are prone to calf cramps, this is the only trimester in which we recommend you focus on strengthening your calves.

How to do it correctly: Place a hardcover book at least 3 inches thick on the floor next to a wall. Stand with your right arm and shoulder nearly touching the wall, and the ball of your right foot on the book. Hold on to the wall for support. Keeping your right knee slightly bent, push up on to the ball of your right foot. Lower to the starting position. Repeat 8 to 12 times, then switch to the left side. Work your way up to three sets.

Things to bear in mind: Press straight up, not off to one side, to target your calf muscles.

To make this move slightly harder: Squeeze your calf muscle at the top of the move. Hold light weights in your hands.

Hamstring and Glute Curl

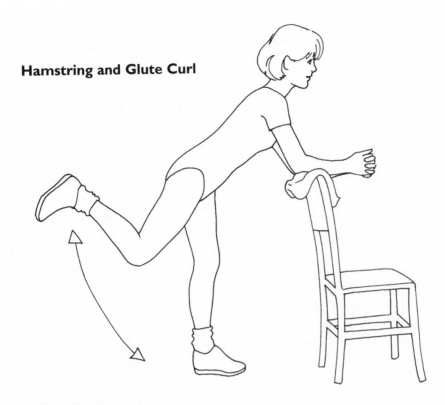

HAMSTRING AND GLUTE CURL

Muscles it targets: Hamstrings and glutes.

Why do it: Strong hamstrings are less prone to injury and, along with strong glutes, they provide a firm base of support for your upper body; weak hamstrings can contribute to lower back pain.

How to do it correctly: Stand 2 to 3 feet away from the rear of a high-backed chair with a towel folded over the top to provide a comfortable resting spot for your arms. Leaning forward from your hips, contract your abdominal muscles and place your forearms on the top of the chairback for support. Keep your left foot flat on the floor and your left knee slightly bent. Reach your right leg behind you with the toe of your right foot resting against the ground. Bending your right knee, lift your right foot toward your butt to the count of two. Lower to the count of two. Exhale as you lift; inhale as you lower. Repeat 8 to 12 times. Switch to the left leg. Work your way up to three sets.

Things to bear in mind: Don't allow your lower back to arch. Keep your hips square.

To make this move slightly harder: Contract your buttocks muscles as you lift. Add leg weights to the working leg.

Plié

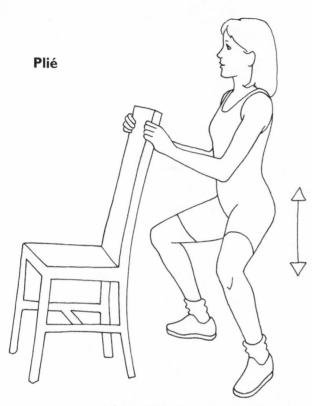

PLIÉ

Muscles it targets: Quadriceps, hamstrings, hip abductors and adductors, and glutes.

Why do it: This move gives you all-purpose leg strength to see you through the upcoming months.

How to do it correctly: Stand with your feet slightly wider than hip-distance apart with your toes turned out gently (to whatever degree feels comfortable), your knees slightly bent, and your abs pulled in firmly. Tuck your butt slightly under to prevent your lower back from arching. Holding on to a chairback for support, bend your knees as far as you can while keeping your spine straight. Hold for a count of two, then straighten. Exhale as you bend; inhale as you straighten. Repeat 8 to 12 times. Work your way up to three sets.

Things to bear in mind: Don't let your knees extend beyond the line of your toes.

To make this move slightly harder: Hold the plié for a count of four before straightening. As you straighten your legs, contract your inner thighs and glutes.

WALL SQUAT

Muscles it targets: Quadriceps, glutes, and abdominals.

Why do it: To firm and strengthen the front of your thighs and train your midsection to hold you upright.

How to do it correctly: Stand with your feet hip-width apart, your abdominals pulled in firmly, and your back resting against a wall. Your feet should be about 18 to 24 inches from the wall. Place your hands on your thighs. Press your hips and lower back into the wall, slide your torso down the wall until your thighs are parallel to the floor. Hold for a count of two. Slide back up to a standing position. Exhale as you bend your legs; inhale as you straighten. Repeat 8 to 12 times. Work your way up to three sets.

Things to bear in mind: Don't bend your knees beyond 90 degrees. Your feet should be far enough from the wall so that when your knees bend, they don't extend beyond your toes.

To make this move slightly harder: Hold weights in your hands.

DUCK SQUAT

Muscles it targets: Oblique abdominals, quadriceps, glutes, and pelvic floor muscles.

Why do it: While it strengthens a number of important muscles, it stretches the muscles of your lower back. It can also be a good preparation for the pushing stage of labor, because it opens your pelvis and takes full advantage of gravity.

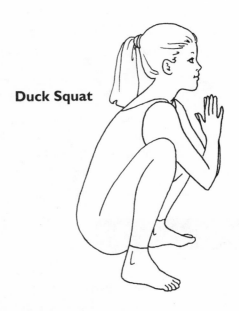

Duck Squat

How to do it correctly: Stand with your feet flat on the floor slightly more than hip-distance apart and your abdominal muscles pulled in firmly. Holding on to a bed frame, heavy couch, or doorknob, gently bend your knees and lower your body into a squatting position. Hold for 15 seconds initially, building up to several minutes if you can. Then lower yourself out of the squat by placing your hands behind you one at a time, and, while you support your weight with your hands, lower your bottom to the floor.

Things to bear in mind: Shift your weight to the outsides of your feet to relieve any pressure on your knees. Keep your heels flat on the floor. (This will get easier the more you do it.)

BASIC KEGEL EXERCISES

Muscles it targets: Pubococcygeus, or PC muscle (see page 16).

Why do it: A strong pelvic floor helps prevent urinary stress incontinence and contributes to stronger orgasms.

How to do it correctly: Start on your hands and knees. Tighten the PC muscle, hold it for 3 seconds, and release. Do 8 to 12 reps. Work your way up to three sets.

Things to bear in mind: Keep breathing as you clench the muscle. To isolate the PC muscle, allow your abdominal and inner thigh muscles to relax.

To make this move slightly harder: While the muscle is clenched, do 5 quick pulses, then release.

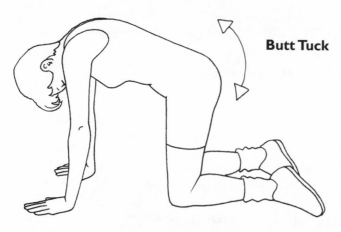

Butt Tuck

BUTT TUCK

Muscles it targets: Glutes.
Why do it: To keep your fanny toned.
How to do it correctly: Start on all fours with your thighs perpendicular to the floor and your back flat. Slowly tuck your tailbone under, squeezing your buttocks together as you tilt your pelvis. Hold for 3 seconds. Return to start. Exhale as you tuck; inhale as you release. Do 8 to 12 reps. Work your way up to three sets.

Things to bear in mind: Don't let your lower back arch when you're in the starting position.

Abdominals

Before performing either of these exercises, check to see if you have a diastasis (see page 30). If you do, substitute the abdominal exercises in chapter 10 for the moves shown here.

BASIC CRUNCH

Muscles it targets: Rectus abdominis.
Why do it: The bigger your belly gets, the weaker these muscles will get, which will place added strain on your back.
How to do it correctly: Lie on a mat on your back with your knees bent and feet flat on the floor, about a foot apart and a comfortable distance from your butt. Keep your heels firmly pressed into the floor to ensure that your abdominals aren't getting any help from your hip flexors (the muscles in front of your hips). Rest your fingertips lightly on the back of your head and keep your elbows out to the sides. As you exhale, raise your head and shoulders off the mat as high as you can. Press your lower back into the floor and pull your abdominal muscles toward your spine as you lift. Hold for a count of two, exhaling as you count. Inhale as you return to the starting position. Repeat 8 to 12 times. Work your way up to three sets.

Things to bear in mind: To keep your head and neck in the proper position, imagine you're holding a tennis ball under your chin.

To make this move slightly harder: Hold the contraction for 2 seconds, then lift your torso slightly higher and hold for another 2 seconds.

CRUNCH WITH ROTATION

Muscles it targets: Obliques and rectus abdominis.

Why do it: Your obliques work with your rectus abdominis and lower back muscles to support your spine, so having strong obliques can help keep lower back pain at bay.

How to do it correctly: Start in the same position as the Basic Crunch (see page 72). When you lift, however, rotate your right shoulder toward your left knee, keeping your hips on the floor. Hold for a count of two, exhaling as you count. Inhale as you lower and repeat with the left shoulder. Do 8 to 12 crunches on each side. Work your way up to three sets.

Things to bear in mind: Be sure to raise your shoulder, not just your elbow. Keep the opposite arm on the floor as you lift.

To make this move slightly harder: Hold the contraction for 2 seconds, then lift your torso slightly higher and hold for another 2 seconds.

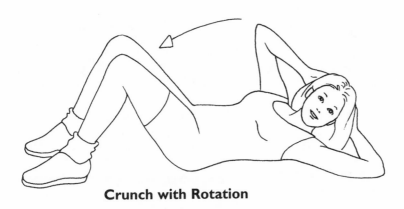

Crunch with Rotation

How to Treat a Sore Muscle

Most minor sprains and strains respond to a combination of rest, ice, compression, and elevation—RICE, for short. If you suffer a minor workout injury, follow this treatment program for at least forty-eight hours after the injury. If pain persists, see your doctor.

• Don't work out for several days to give your body time to recuperate.

• Ice the painful area as soon as you can to reduce the swelling, and reapply an ice pack for 15 to 20 minutes three or four times a day. Ice also deadens the pain by constricting blood flow to the area.

• Wrap an Ace bandage around the area to keep the swelling down. It should be snug but not so tight that your limb goes numb.

• Elevating the injured area reduces the swelling by encouraging the fluid buildup to drain off. Elevation alone won't do much good, but when used in conjunction with the preceding suggestions, it can help you get back on your feet.

Enhancing Flexibility

Like flossing your teeth and checking your breasts for lumps, stretching is something you know you *should* do. But let's be honest: When you're short on time, feeling tired, or running low on motivation (all of which apply right now, no doubt) you skip it, right? You're not alone. For most people, stretching is the component of the fitness triad most likely to be neglected, probably because it's the least sexy.

Both cardiovascular and strength training hold out the promise of a better body by helping you burn fat or build muscle. If you do them over time, they'll enhance your physique in some real, tangible ways—you'll drop a dress size, say, or look better in your old jeans. Stretching can't make that claim. Although there are plenty of books and videos that have tried to sell the stretch-your-way-to-a-better-body concept, the truth is the benefits of stretching are less visual and more anatomical. In other words, it may not help you slip into that little black maternity smock you've got your eye on, but it will improve your health and well-being—especially now that you're pregnant—so it's just as important as the other parts of your fitness regimen.

Stretching can mean the difference between residing in a comfortable body that moves with grace and fluidity or one that clicks, creaks, cracks, and groans with every movement. It can counteract some notorious markers of aging, like an aching back, painful knees, rounded shoulders, and easily pulled muscles. And if that isn't enough, here's one of its most powerful hidden selling points: It has the ability to ease muscle tension and slough off stress and anxiety, keeping you centered both physically and emotionally.

Why is stretching so important now? During pregnancy, when your body is pulled and distended in unimaginable ways, stretching can go a long way toward keeping you flexible in the truest sense of the word—better able to go with the flow, adapt to the onslaught of postural and muscular changes, readjust, realign, rejuvenate. It's the only way to lengthen the muscles that will start getting shorter and tighter as your pregnancy progresses, including the ones in your lower back, your chest, your thighs, and your hips. Later on, stretching can help prevent painful middle-of-the-night calf cramps. And, throughout your pregnancy, it will help you move with more freedom and stay active by keeping your muscles, joints, tendons, and ligaments as supple and pain-free as possible.

Sound convincing? Good. Here's the best part: Stretching doesn't require a bit of time commitment because it doesn't have to be done in a single, daily session to be beneficial. Although it's helpful to do a few stretches after you exercise so your muscles don't become too tight, you can steal quiet moments to limber up throughout the day—when you're in the shower, on the phone, waiting in line at the deli, even driving your car. To help you get into the habit of incorporating stretching into your daily routine as well as after your workout, we offer suggestions for when and where to do each of the moves in our flexibility routine. As you become more accustomed to stretching, you'll find more and more ways to sneak it into your life. And by the way, if you *do* have a chunk of time to devote to flexibility, or if you simply aren't up to a cardio or strength workout but want to do *something,* our head-to-toe routine is not only a comprehensive, effective way to work the kinks out but also a safe, simple way to achieve a minimum level of exercise benefit.

As with everything else when you're pregnant, there are some rules you should abide by to stretch safely while still getting the most out of each effort:

• **Be aware** that you're operating under the influence of hormones. That means your body's tendons and ligaments are looser and your joints are less stable than normal, so you need to approach stretching with more care and finesse than usual. If you're superlimber (if you cruised through our stretching tests in chapter 2 like a contortionist), you run the risk of overstretching like never before. To be sure you don't exceed the safety zone, don't push your stretches to the limit. With every stretch you should feel like you could go a little bit farther—just don't do it.

• **Breathe slowly and easily** through every stretch. Inhale through your nose and exhale through your mouth. If you are bending forward to stretch, exhale as you bend and breathe slowly as you hold the posture. The idea is to be relaxed, and one way to do that is to breathe naturally.

• **Stretch with awareness.** You should feel a slight tension, *not pain,* in the first few seconds of the stretch that diminishes once you've held it for 5 to 10 seconds. If a move is painful or the tension doesn't diminish, back off.

• **Hold each stretch** for about 20 to 30 seconds, except for ones in which you do repetitions.

- **Don't bounce.** You can actually harm your muscles and make them *tighter* by forcing a stretch with ballistic movements.

HEAD BOB

Muscles it targets: Neck and upper back.

Why do it: To ease neck tension and promote upper-body postural awareness.

How to do it correctly: While standing or sitting cross-legged, tilt your head slowly to the right, so your right ear drops toward your right shoulder. Return to center. Repeat to the left. Repeat 5 times. Then bring your chin toward your chest and return to center. Repeat 5 times.

When to do it: In the shower with the warm water running on your neck, at your desk, when you're watching television.

UPPER BODY STRETCH

Muscles it targets: Traps, rhomboids, and delts.

Why do it: To lengthen the muscles in your shoulders and upper back, release tension, and counteract bad posture.

How to do it correctly: While standing or sitting cross-legged, raise your arms out in front of you to shoulder height and interlace your fingers so your palms are facing away from your body. Press forward through the palms and hold the stretch. Then exhale as you slowly raise your arms up over your head, keeping your elbows soft. Taking care not to arch your back, straighten your elbows, pressing your palms toward the ceiling. Hold the stretch.

When to do it: When you first wake up in the morning, when you're sitting at your desk, when you're standing in a line.

CHEST STRETCH

Muscles it targets: Pecs and delts.

Why do it: To open up your chest area and combat rounded shoulders.

How to do it correctly: While standing or sitting cross-legged, interlace your hands behind your back. Lift your arms gently up and back, allowing your shoulders to fall open as you do so. Keep your chin tucked in. Hold the stretch.

When to do it: Anytime you feel yourself slumping forward, particularly when you're sitting at your desk, washing dishes, or watching television.

SIDE STRETCH

Muscles it targets: Triceps, obliques, and lats.

Why do it: To maintain flexibility in your trunk.

How to do it correctly: While standing or sitting cross-legged, reach your right arm straight up toward the ceiling, pulling out of your waist. Hold for 3 seconds. Repeat on your left side. Repeat 5 times with each arm. Then, with your right arm reaching overhead again, place your left hand on your left hip and bend your waist slightly to the left to increase the stretch on the right side. Hold for 3 seconds and repeat on the left side. Repeat 5 times.

When to do it: After your shower, when you're watching television, after a workout.

SEATED HAMSTRING STRETCH

Muscles it targets: Hamstrings.

Why do it: To relieve lower back pain and tension.

How to do it correctly: Sit on the floor with your right leg out in front of you and your left leg bent so your left foot rests against your right inner thigh. (If you need to, sit with your back against a wall for support.) Adjust your posture so you're sitting squarely on both hips. Loop a towel or sweatshirt around your right heel, maintaining slight tension by pulling back on it with your arms. Press forward through your right heel and lean slightly forward from your hips until you feel a gentle stretch in your hamstring. Hold the stretch. Repeat on the left side.

When to do it: After you exercise, when you're watching television, after a long day of standing or sitting.

Seated Hamstring Stretch

HIP CIRCLES

Muscles it targets: Lower back, abdominals, and hips.

Why do it: To release tension in your lower back and ease pelvic congestion.

How to do it correctly: Stand with your feet about hip-distance apart and your abdominal muscles pulled in firmly. With your hands on your hips, gently move your hips left, forward, right, and back so you make a fluid circle. Rotate 5 times slowly to the right. Then reverse the direction.

When to do it: In the shower, while you're stirring food on the stove, after a run or walk.

QUADRICEPS STRETCH

Muscles it targets: Quadriceps.

Why do it: To prevent pulled muscles when you're active.

How to do it correctly: Holding on to the back of a chair or wall with your right hand for support, bring your left foot up behind you, grab your toes with your left hand, and pull the foot toward your butt. Bend your supporting leg slightly and keep your pelvis tucked under. (Don't arch your back or lean forward.) Hold the stretch. Repeat with the right leg.

When to do it: After you do your preworkout warm-up, after you work out, when you're standing in a line, when you're cooking.

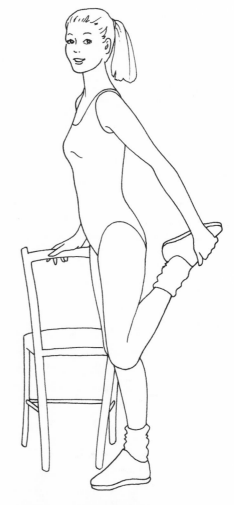

Quadriceps Stretch

INNER THIGH STRETCH

Muscles it targets: Adductors, or inner thigh muscles.

Why do it: To keep the upper leg and pelvic area limber.

How to do it correctly: Stand with your legs 4 feet apart. Keeping your left foot facing forward, turn your right foot out about 45 degrees. Then bend your right leg and lunge slightly to the right, until you feel a stretch in your left inner thigh. Don't let your right knee extend beyond the toes of your right foot. If you don't feel enough of a stretch, spread your legs farther apart. Hold the stretch. Repeat on the other side.

When to do it: After you do your preworkout warm-up, after you work out, when you're standing in a line, when you're cooking.

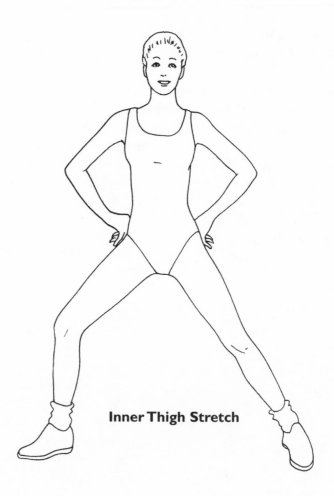

Inner Thigh Stretch

Calf and Achilles Stretch

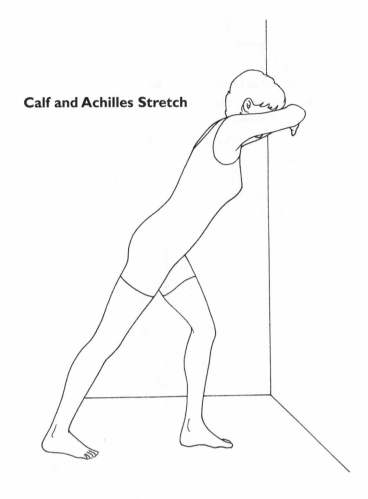

CALF AND ACHILLES STRETCH

Muscles it targets: The muscles in your calf.

Why do it: To make walking, running, and jumping easier, to prevent injuries, and to prevent cramping.

How to do it correctly: Face a wall and place your forearms against it, shoulder-width apart. Bend your left leg and step back with your right leg. Both feet should be flat on the floor with your toes pointing forward. Allow your weight to fall forward onto your arms until you feel a stretch in the calf of the right leg. Hold the stretch. Repeat on the other side. Then, with your right leg in the rear again, bend both legs with your weight forward against the wall until you feel a stretch in your right Achilles tendon. Hold the stretch. Repeat on the other side.

When to do it: After you do your preworkout warm-up, after you work out.

POSTURE ADJUSTER

Muscles it targets: Your whole body. It doesn't stretch your muscles so much as bring them into alignment.

Why do it: To enhance your balance and correct your posture.

How to do it correctly: Start in a comfortable standing position, holding on to a wall for support. Then bring your right foot up so the sole of the foot is resting on your left inner thigh. With your right knee pointing out to the side, press your right foot and your left thigh together to relieve pressure on your back. If you can, bring your hands together in a praying position. (Gazing at a fixed point will help you keep your balance.) If not, continue holding on to the wall. Hold for 15 seconds. Repeat on the other side.

When to do it: After a long day, when you're stressed out, at the end of a workout.

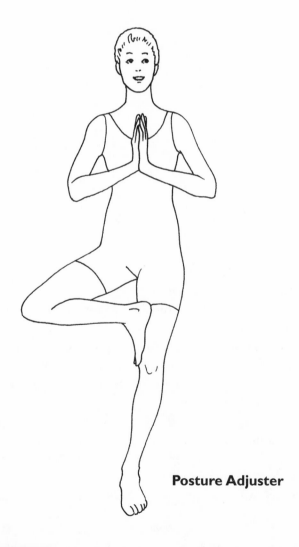

Posture Adjuster

ANKLE WARM-UPS

Muscles it targets: The muscles, tendons, and ligaments surrounding your ankle.

Why do it: To prevent strains and sprains and maintain strength and coordination in your ankles.

How to do it correctly: Holding on to the back of a chair or wall with your left hand for support, lift your right leg slightly (in front of you) and circle the ankle to the right 5 times. Then circle it to the left. Repeat with the other leg.

When to do it: When you first get out of bed in the morning, when you're standing in line, when you're talking on the phone.

THE
second trimester

Your Changing Body

Cardiovascular Fitness

Getting Stronger

Enhancing Flexibility

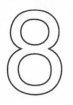

Your Changing Body

You're out of your first trimester, and we'd like to take this moment to breathe a collective sigh of relief . . . whew. Now is the time when most women start feeling less like guinea pigs for some diabolical science experiment and more like real, honest-to-goodness human beings. The debilitating nausea and sluggishness of early pregnancy should be easing up along with your fears of miscarriage. Also, your frame of mind is probably better now that you feel more like yourself, and the initial, often rocky emotional adjustment to life as a human incubator may be giving way to a pleasant sense of excitement and anticipation. All of this means your fitness forecast is looking bright.

For those of you who did little but shuffle around the house in slippers and a bathrobe for the first twelve weeks, cheer up. It's not too late to start an exercise program. In fact, there's never been a better time to slip into a little sweat-friendly gear (whatever still fits) and take your new body for a test drive. Of course, as you start looking more visibly pregnant, which will happen any day now, there are a number of additional factors you're going to have to take into consideration when you head out to exercise.

Postural changes If your bearing wasn't exactly statuesque before pregnancy, it certainly won't be improved by your increasingly apparent abdominal bulge. Even the most dancerlike bodies are thrown out of alignment by the added weight of midpregnancy. Here's what's happening: As your uterus grows, your center of gravity begins to shift, pulling the top of your pelvis forward. As your pelvis tilts, the natural curve in your lower back starts to increase, and a condition known as *lordosis,* or swayback, sets in. Meanwhile, to counterbalance the exaggerated dip of your lower back, you may allow your shoulders to slump and your head to jut forward, all of which results in posture that looks, well, schlumpy.

How to Cope with Gestational Diabetes

Sometime between your twenty-fourth and twenty-eighth week of pregnancy, your doctor is going to ask you to go to a medical lab before you've eaten anything in the morning and drink a special glucose solution that tastes sweet and syrupy. This is called a glucose screening test. After an hour, a lab technician will draw a blood sample to check your blood sugar level in response to the sugary concoction.

Most women's bodies respond to this test by producing more insulin, a hormone that regulates the amount of glucose in your blood. Some women, however, may not be able to produce enough insulin at one time to handle the increase in blood sugar, or they may be unable to use the insulin they do produce efficiently; either way, the results indicate gestational diabetes, a condition affecting fewer than 3 percent of pregnant women. The most common result of gestational diabetes is an extralarge baby (and possibly a cesarean delivery), because the baby receives extra glucose through the placenta. Fortunately, doctors say it's fairly simple to keep gestational diabetes under control.

• Heed your doctor's special dietary advice. Women with gestational diabetes typically are put on a 2,000- to 2,200-calorie-a-day diet that contains almost no simple carbohydrates.

• Get daily exercise. The second line of treatment for gestational diabetes is exercise, which lowers your body's glucose levels. Shoot for a 20-minute walk or swim daily to keep blood sugar levels under control.

• Be conscientious about self-testing your blood sugar levels. The blood test usually involves a simple fingertip prick so you can test your blood with a blood glucose meter. Fifteen to 30 percent of women with gestational diabetes will also need to give themselves insulin injections two or three times a day to keep their blood glucose levels under control.

But your appearance isn't the only thing that will suffer. Allowing your pelvis to tilt forward on a daily basis causes your abdominal muscles to stretch and weaken and the muscles of your lower back to shorten and tighten, which makes the curve in your lower back even deeper. And if that isn't bad enough, this posture–related muscle imbalance can cause backaches and muscle spasms, both of which can make you feel lousy and put a serious crimp in your exercise program.

Now for the good news: Although these postural changes are perfectly natural, they're not inevitable (or permanent) if you know what's happening and make the effort to correct them—which we suggest you start doing *pronto*. First, do a quick posture check. Stand in front of a mirror. Now turn sideways. Just stand normally. (No fair adjusting anything.) How do you look? Is your head sitting atop your shoulders or sticking out in front of them? Are your shoulders in line with your hips and knees or are they drooping forward? Is your lower back only slightly curved, or does it look like you could balance a can of soda on your butt?

Now pull yourself into proper alignment. When you look at yourself from the side, your ear, shoulder, hip, knee, and ankle should form a straight line. To get there, you need to rock your pelvis back into the proper position under your ribs (it will feel like you're tucking your butt slightly under), pull your chin in so it sits above the notch between your collarbones, and allow your shoulders to relax into a more upright position. (Don't forcibly pull your shoulders back into a militaristic stance. That will only throw your lower back off again.)

Switch back and forth between your usual (bad) posture and the correct posture to get a sense of how the two feel. Then remind yourself throughout the day to stand up straight. (This is actually good practice for motherhood.) Once you get in the proper-posture habit, you'll find that you won't tire as easily, and you'll move with more grace and agility, both of which, incidentally, will serve you well as you work out.

Loosening joints and ligaments in your pelvis The pubic bone is actually made up of two separate bones joined together in the middle of the pubic area by a strong ligament. Under the influence of relaxin, a hormone released in increasingly greater amounts throughout pregnancy, this ligament can become so soft and unstable that the two bones may literally separate. It sounds bad, but this phenomenon is actually desirable, because it increases the dimensions of your pelvis and creates more room for your baby to pass through the birth canal during childbirth.

Be warned, however: A number of pesky ailments can also crop up as a result of this pelvic shift. In fact, if you're starting to feel funny little pains on the edges of your pelvis, you're already experiencing one of the most common side effects: round ligament pain. Ranging anywhere from mildly cramplike to sharp and stabbing, round ligament pain is usually worst when you get out of bed or up from a chair. Rest will generally alleviate the pain and learning the correct way to get up from a sitting or lying-down position can help you avoid the problem. To stand up from a chair, put your hands on your legs just above your knees, lean forward, and push yourself up slowly with your arms. To lie down, or to stand up after lying down, roll over onto one hip and use your arms to lower or lift your body.

For particularly annoying cases, try the following exercise, which was shown by researchers at Case Western Reserve University in Cleveland,

Ohio, to be effective in relieving both the intensity and duration of round ligament pain: Stand barefoot with your feet together, one hand holding the back of a chair or touching a wall for support. Keeping both legs straight, raise your right leg up by lifting your right hip so your right foot is about 2 inches off the floor. Keep your shoulders and the bottom of your right foot parallel to the floor. Hold the right leg in the air for 6 seconds, then lower. Repeat 10 times on the right, then switch to the left. This movement tilts your hip and pelvis about 30 degrees, which releases and relaxes the irritated ligament.

A small number of women have a large degree of pelvic separation, which can cause severe pain in the center of the pubic area, a condition known as pubic symphysis pain. This type of pain is usually exacerbated by activities in which your legs move separately, such as when you use a stair-climbing machine, walk, or do the flutter kick in swimming. If any exercise causes pain along the midline of your pubic area, stop and switch to another type of exercise, like a rowing machine, in which your legs work in unison.

Scientists believe relaxin affects your pelvis more than other joints in your body, but it's likely that it has at least a minimal effect on all your joints, making them less stable and predisposing them to injury and dislocation. That's why doctors say you should try to avoid sports that involve sudden stops and direction changes, such as tennis and racquetball. Instead, run, walk, and bike on smooth, even surfaces and take extra precautions like lowering the height of the step in step aerobics classes. (See "Sports You Can Do," page 62, for other suggestions.)

Diastasis In chapter 1, we told you a little about this condition, in which the two halves of your vertical abdominal muscles separate slightly, but it typically doesn't set in until the second trimester, when your expanding uterus starts exerting more pressure from the inside on these outermost muscles. Although there's nothing serious about this condition, if you have it you should modify certain exercise moves and be religious about strengthening your abdominal muscles. (To perform a simple diastasis check, see our instructions on page 30.)

During the day, as you go about your daily chores, pretend you're wearing a skimpy bikini on a crowded beach to help you remember to suck in your gut. It sounds goofy, but even this simple effort can build a stronger midsection, which can combat some of the abdominal laxity diastasis causes. Pay special attention to pulling in your abdomen when you move in ways that can stress those muscles, like when you're getting out of a chair or even lifting a gallon of milk off the top shelf of your refrigerator.

How to Cope with Swelling

Puffy. The word takes on new meaning right about now. As many as 75 percent of pregnant women develop some mild swelling, especially in their ankles and feet. Often worse in warm weather and late in the day, particularly if you've been on your feet a lot, pregnancy edema can most likely be blamed on the onslaught of extra fluids circulating in your system now. There's more blood, more amniotic fluid, more plain old H_2O.

Although the bottom parts of your body—your feet and ankles—are usually hardest hit by water retention, your hands and even your face can blow up from time to time. That's why a lot of women remove their wedding rings midpregnancy—better to take them off now than to have them cut off (cringe) later.

Usually, a little swelling is nothing to worry about. But if your hands or face become more than a little puffy or if the swelling doesn't go away with a good night's rest, you should call your doctor. Swelling can sometimes signal the onset of preeclampsia, or pregnancy-induced hypertension.

To minimize the irritation factor of everyday swelling, heed these beat-the-bloat pointers:

• Make sure your shoes fit. Partly from the swelling and partly from a natural spreading of your foot joints, your shoes may be suddenly snug. (For suggestions on buying new workout shoes, see "Fit Your Feet," page 95.)

• Don't stand for long periods of time, and don't sit for long periods without taking a move-around break.

• Elevate your legs every chance you get.

• When you can, lie down on your left side, which helps your body keep the fluids moving through your system. Here's why: The vena cava, the large vein that brings blood back from your lower body to your heart, lies behind and slightly to the right of your uterus, so when you lie on your left side, you're actually giving that vein a little more room in which to work. That doesn't mean it's dangerous to lie on your right side, but resting on your left side is just slightly more conducive to optimal blood flow.

• Avoid socks or stockings with tourniquet-like elastic.

Weight gain By now your appetite is what many health care practitioners euphemistically call "hearty." Insatiable is more like it. Especially if you spent the better part of the first trimester struggling to eat enough, you now probably find yourself fighting the urge to eat too much. Try to focus on consuming a wide variety of healthful foods and maintain a regular exercise routine, and your weight gain shouldn't get too out of hand.

Bitter as this pill may be to swallow, you need to keep in mind that weight gain goes with the territory. (Even hot-shot celebrities haven't figured out how to stay skinny *during* pregnancy.) Most doctors say you should be putting on about a pound a week now. That means your body is going to go from pleasantly plump to really round during these next few months, a change that can be alarming to even the most contented mother-to-be. But what's happening inside you is even more extraordinary. Your baby, which entered its fourth month as a 2- to 3-inch being, will measure somewhere in the 11- to 14-inch range by the end of this trimester. Imagine the kind of energy it takes to grow 8 or more inches in three months! No wonder you're ravenous.

If you gained a lot of weight during the first trimester, you're going to notice even more significant changes every time you look in a mirror, or, worse yet, see a picture of your prepregnancy self. There's no way to get those early pounds off now, so it's best to resign yourself to a little extra padding and get on with the business of having a healthy, happy, *active* pregnancy.

If you're really struggling with the body-image issue, here's a trick that will help you see your pregnant form from a new point of view: Surround yourself with beautiful pictures of pregnant women. The famous *Vanity Fair* cover featuring Demi Moore comes to mind (you can make a color photocopy of it at the library), but there also are a number of greeting cards and books that show pregnant women looking everything from radiant to glamorous to downright sexy. Post a few of those photos on your refrigerator or bathroom mirror so you're confronted with images of maternal beauty daily, and you just may begin to see your own body for the wonder it is.

Fitness Q & A

My exercise tights are snug at the waist. Is it safe to wear them?

You're probably not going to harm the baby by wearing exercise gear that's on the small side, but if you are prone to varicose veins or you have a family history of them, restrictive clothing can make them more likely to occur. Moreover, there are a couple of other really good reasons to invest in some better-fitting gear (or at least steal some baggy sweatpants from your husband's closet). First, although you probably don't need us to tell you this, it's uncomfortable to wear pants that are too tight, particularly when you're going to be sweating in them. You probably have enough niggling aches and pains right now. Why add this discomfort to your woes? Second, looser clothing will allow air to circulate around your body more freely, which will help you keep cooler. Although the temperature factor isn't as much of a concern once you're in the second trimester, you still want to stay as cool during exercise as you can. Besides, a number of maternity lines have really cute, comfortable clothing designed especially for exercising pregnant women, and there's nothing like a little retail therapy to give your attitude a boost. Buy a few new items now, and you're sure to get a lot of use out of them in the coming months.

I've heard that I shouldn't lift anything heavier than about 10 pounds. Is that true?

Stash this one in your old wives' tales file. Sure, if you are having a high-risk pregnancy of some sort, your doctor may restrict your lifting. But in a normal pregnancy, you should be able to lift a reasonable amount of weight—a small child, say, or a bag of groceries. Just be sure you lift the correct way: Kneel down before you lift so the muscles of your legs, not your back, bear the brunt of the weight, pull in your abdominal muscles as you lift, and hold the "package" close to your body to avoid straining your back. If you're lifting weights, be sure you continue to breathe throughout the movement, exhaling as you lift and inhaling as you lower the weight to its starting position.

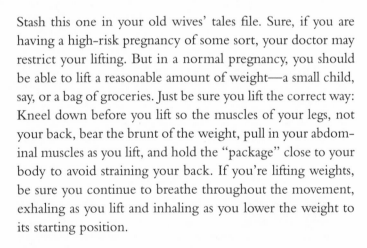

I ran throughout the first trimester, but now that my belly extends past my pubic bones, it feels sort of funny. Can I continue?

The simple answer is yes, as long as you have your doctor's okay and you're not experiencing anything unusual, like pelvic pain or knee problems. You're not going to jounce the baby loose or upset the little critter with the motion. The more complicated response requires a little self-examination:

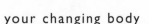

If it feels funny, why would you want to continue doing it? Although running is a perfectly wonderful form of exercise, there are lots of other ways to get a workout that might feel better to your body, such as walking, swimming, and bicycling. Why not try one of them for a day or two (or check out our running/walking program, page 60) and then decide if you really want to continue with your usual routine?

 I took a racquetball in the stomach during a recent game. Could it have injured the baby?

Probably not. By about the twelfth week of pregnancy, your uterus rises high enough above the level of the pubic bone that it can be seen and felt by your doctor. Once this happens, the chance of injury to your uterus caused by a direct blow increases, but it's still highly unlikely. Injury to the baby, who is well protected by a cushioning of amniotic fluid, is even less likely. Still, that's one of the reasons many doctors say you should avoid sports like racquetball that could involve a direct blow to the abdomen. If you notice any unusual symptoms—bleeding, say, or abdominal cramping—call your doctor immediately.

Fit Your Feet

Been a size 7 narrow all your life? Don't be surprised if your feet expand right along with the rest of you. Several factors contribute to your changing shoe size: swelling, which is temporary, weight gain (yes, you can get fat feet), and spreading joints, which may be permanent. You might be able to squeeze into a too-small shoe to do chores around the house (although why you would want to is beyond us), but you should definitely have properly fitting footwear for athletic activities like walking and running, because sore feet and blisters will sideline you for days or even weeks.

If you've shopped for new athletic shoes anytime in the past ten years or so, you know there's enough sales jargon to make you feel like you were shopping for a nuclear reactor instead of a sports shoe. Marketing speak aside, athletic shoes for different sports *are* different. Here's how to cut through all the muck and pick a shoe that's right for your sport.

Walking shoes should have a flexible forefoot. To test this out, grab the shoe at the heel and toe and bend it. A good walking shoe will flex easily to a 45-degree angle in the ball of the foot, not the arch. Now, twist the shoe as if you were wringing out a wet rag. It should be flexible, because when you walk you actually place your weight on your little toe first and roll slightly inward. Finally, put the shoe on a flat surface and, with a pencil, push down on the toe. The heel should lift off the ground. In fact, the more lift, the more spring the shoe will give your stride. A good shoe also has a low rounded or beveled heel to facilitate the natural heel-to-toe roll that happens in a good walking stride and a simple upper portion of the shoe, preferably made of a breathable, lightweight mesh or synthetic fabric, not leather.

Aerobics shoes should have good ankle support (although not as much as you'd find in basketball shoes) and plenty of cushioning in the ball of the foot—enough so that when you walk in them you have that I-never-want-to-take-these-shoes-off feeling.

Running shoes should flex in the ball of the foot when you bend them, but they should give only to about 30 degrees. A good running shoe should be cushioned but not so much so that you can't feel your foot hitting the ground. (Be sure to test this.) Look for stable heel counters. You don't want your foot sliding around as you run.

No matter what type of shoe you need, you should follow these basic principles:
• Shop in late afternoon, when your feet are likely to be at their puffiest.
• Wear or bring along a pair of athletic socks.
• Make sure there's at least one thumb's width of space between the end of your big toe and the tip of the shoe.
• Take your top contenders for a spin down the pavement outside the store. If the proprietors won't indulge this test, shop elsewhere.

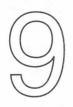

Cardiovascular Fitness

If you haven't been exercising up to this point, now is the hour. Physical changes will be coming at a fast and furious pace for the next few months, but exercise will keep you ahead of the curve, so to speak, by helping you stay in touch with your changing shape and fend off a variety of common pregnancy afflictions, from backaches to body-image problems. Since you're probably feeling better physically, you may be ready to really attack your workouts. Don't overdo it. All the original pregnancy precautions still apply (see "The Seven Commandments of Pregnancy Fitness," page 52), and as your belly expands—which happens this trimester in a big way—we're going to add some new ones.

The first new warning: Watch your step. Think the word *klutz* could never apply to you? You've never been pregnant before. Even the most graceful creatures find themselves becoming just a tad clumsier during this trimester (and even more so next trimester). You'll drop things more often. You'll graze the doorway as you walk from room to room instead of swooshing through it as you used to do. And, if you're physically active, you may twist an ankle, misjudge the height of a step or curb, or simply feel less capable and in control than you're accustomed to feeling.

There are a couple of reasons for this sudden spaz attack. First, the pregnancy hormone relaxin is allowing your ligaments, especially those in your pelvis, to loosen, which means your joints aren't as stable as they once were. Second, your balance is just starting to be thrown out of whack now that your breasts are larger and your belly is protruding from the front of your body like a newly formed appendage. Just as awkwardness often accompanies the adolescent growth spurt, it can be part of the pregnancy expansion as well.

The second word of warning: Keep your intensity level moderate, even if that means you're going slower than you were a month ago. This isn't a contest. You need to let go of any preconceived notions of what you "should" be able to do and replace them with reality-based goals of what you *are* able to do. If you haven't been using the talk test or the Rate of Perceived Exertion (RPE) scale, start. And you may want to begin monitoring your heart rate as well, as long as you don't use it as the sole guide to your exertion. (See chapter 2 for how to find your heart rate as well as the heart rate range some researchers feel is safe during pregnancy.)

Although different women respond to the physical changes of pregnancy in different ways, you should expect the extra pounds and funky weight distribution to begin to cut into your stamina at least slightly. According to the American College of Obstetricians and Gynecologists (ACOG), most women who perform regular weight-bearing exercise prior to pregnancy notice a progressive decline in performance beginning in the early months. In one study involving runners, aerobic dancers, and cross-country skiers, 60 percent noted significantly decreased exercise performance in early pregnancy and more than 50 percent had voluntarily cut out exercise completely by the third trimester. Only 10 percent of the women in the study maintained their performance at or near preconception levels throughout pregnancy. In another study of well-conditioned runners, overall performance decreased by about 10 percent in early pregnancy followed by a gradual decline to roughly 50 percent of preconception levels by early in the third trimester.

Which brings us to our third warning: Replace activities that feel "wrong" with ones that feel "right." Some women may never have this awareness. Others find that high-impact activities like running fall into the former category and that low- or nonimpact exercise falls into the latter. Some studies suggest that women who begin various forms of non-weight-bearing exercise like cycling or swimming in early pregnancy are able to maintain a high-intensity, moderate-duration training regimen throughout the third trimester. Those findings, when combined with the ones on high-impact activities mentioned above, led the ACOG study to conclude that "the maternal adaptation to both physiologic and morphologic [physical] changes appears to favor non-weight-bearing exercise over weight-bearing exercise during pregnancy." That doesn't mean if you're a running freak you have to hang up your shoes until after pregnancy, just that the pregnant body may be better suited to other activities. It's something to think about.

How to Cope with Dizziness

From the moment you found out you were pregnant, you've felt like you were riding a Tilt-a-Whirl of crazy emotions. But that woozy, lurching feeling that just set in recently has a real biological cause: the pressure of your expanding uterus on your blood vessels.

Dizziness most commonly occurs when you stand up fast. Called postural hypotension, this kind of dizziness is caused by the blood rushing out of your head and into your extremities, a change that, not surprisingly, leaves you feeling light-headed. Another frequent cause of dizziness is low blood sugar, which can occur when you go too long without food (yet another reason why restricting your food intake is a very bad idea). Not surprisingly, this may be particularly prevalent in pregnant women who exercise, because they're burning calories faster than sedentary women and, therefore, need more fuel to maintain an adequate concentration of glucose in their blood.

The best way to handle a dizzy spell is to lie down, which will increase the circulation to your brain. If you can, elevate your feet. If you're not in a place where you can lie down, sit and put your head between your knees until the feeling passes. To prevent an occurrence:

• Always get up slowly. Don't rush to answer the phone or the doorbell. A couple of seconds more could mean the difference between rising safely and landing right back on your butt.

• Don't skip meals, especially breakfast. You need a steady intake of calories, particularly protein and carbohydrates, to keep your blood sugar level on an even keel.

• Keep snacks handy. You can battle that vertiginous feeling by gobbling up a handful of raisins, a piece of fruit, or a few crackers.

• Get some fresh air. Close, overheated quarters can make even the most stoic pregnant woman feel queasy. If you start feeling closed-in, get out.

Our fourth and final second-trimester caution: Remember that you're not exercising to lose weight, you're exercising to stay healthy. We know we've mentioned this before, but it bears repeating now that your shape is noticeably changing. We'd rather have you sit out the entire pregnancy than fight every single pound as if it were a sign of inadequacy or failure.

The bottom line here, as usual, is that you need to use your common sense. Be careful. Move more slowly. Pay attention to your body. Pretend you're taking care of a child rather than your grown-up self, and you have to look at every activity with a newly critical eye to be sure it's safe for this somewhat-altered being you have become.

Get in Touch with Your Changing Shape

To get more in touch with how your ever-changing body feels, try this routine that borrows its introspective point of view from mindfulness meditation. Choose a clear, safe path that you know well. It can be in your living room or in a park. The point is to find a place that is obstacle-free, so you can focus your attention inward rather than outward. Walk slowly on the path, paying close attention to the way your body feels as it moves. Focus on your feet touching the ground, the weight transfer as you shift your body forward, your posture, the way your arms swing. Do your feet feel like they strike the ground at a slightly different angle now? Does your walking posture feel more rounded and hunched? Do your hips have a slightly unhinged feeling? By getting used to these changes in slow motion, you can move more safely and with greater awareness when you pick up the pace.

Guidelines for New Exercisers

If you're just getting on board with the exercise program, fear not. You can still reap many of the benefits of pregnancy fitness as long as you follow a safe, effective start-up regimen. (See chapter 5 for some important information on your mind-set.) Because it's more important to exercise regularly (at least three days a week) than to exercise for a long period of time, we recommend that you ease into a program by doing the easiest cardiovascular activity you can do *every day*. For most people, the simplest, least-likely-to-be-blown-off type of exercise is walking, because you can do it anywhere—inside a mall, on a path through the woods, even on a crowded, urban sidewalk. Based on that fact, here's our suggestion: Get into the habit of walking at least 10 minutes every day for at least two weeks. Then, follow one of our two beginner programs in chapter 5.

Guidelines for Intermediate and Advanced Exercisers

By now you probably have a pretty good sense of your body's evolving (or devolving) capabilities, but you may very well be battling the boredom beast if you've been dedicated to one routine for the past several months. Our cross-training program in chapter 5 is always a good option for women who are interested in a broad range of activities, but for those of you who are into swimming or walking, we've created two fresh routines that will not only breathe new life into your workout but also address your unique physical needs this trimester.

Swimming Our first trimester program incorporated a kickboard into the routine, because our focus was on building leg strength to prepare for the added weight of later pregnancy. Now is the time to add an upper body component, however, because the weaker your abs get, the more strain your upper body is going to suffer during even the simplest tasks—pulling plates out of the cupboard, lifting your body from the bed, pushing the vacuum around the living room. To give your upper body a better water workout, we've added some laps using a pull-buoy, a foam gadget you hold between your thighs as you swim. As always, pay attention to your intensity level, rest if you feel winded, and stop as soon as you feel fatigue setting in.

the program: Swim 5 to 10 minutes at an easy pace to warm up. Then swim 100 yards at a brisk pace. You should feel like you're working somewhat hard. Swim with a kickboard for 200 yards. Rest 2 minutes. (If you get too tired, rest after the first 100 yards, then continue.) Swim at a brisk pace for 300 yards. Rest 3 minutes. Swim with the kickboard for 100 yards. Rest 3 minutes. Swim with the pull-buoy between your legs for 150 yards. Rest 1 minute. Swim 50 yards at an easy pace to cool down. Note: If you are experiencing pain at the edges of your pelvis, try swimming more laps with the pull-buoy and eliminate the kickboard work.

Walking If you still enjoy running, feel free to continue that workout, or try our running/walking program in chapter 5. But if you've already committed to walking, you can continue to challenge your heart with our interval walking program, in which you alternate short, moderately intense bursts of walking with periods of relatively easy walking. Professional athletes use this speed-it-up-slow-it-down approach for extra conditioning, but it can work for anyone who is interested in building or maintaining cardiovascular fitness.

the program: Start by walking 5 minutes at an easy pace to warm up. Then walk for 10 minutes at your usual, fairly brisk pace. For the next 16 minutes alternate 1-minute periods of fast walking with 3-minute periods of easy to moderate walking. If you get so winded during the fast-walking periods that you can't catch your breath during the subsequent easy periods, turn your pace down a notch. Cool down by walking 5 minutes at an easy pace.

How to Cope with Varicose Veins

Plump legs are one thing, but ones with bulgy blue veins are really too much of an injustice. Still, that lovely condition known as varicose veins is something that as many as 40 percent of pregnant women have to put up with.

Varicose veins occur when a combination of pregnancy hormones and increased blood volume causes the blood vessel walls to stretch so much that the valves normally preventing blood backflow don't close properly. As a result, blood pools in the veins, making them distended. In women who are prone to the condition, which is hereditary, varicose veins often appear for the first time during pregnancy. They can cause anything from mild achiness to severe pain, and can produce what looks like a topographical road map from your ankle to thigh. They usually disappear after you've had the baby, but they may be worse in subsequent pregnancies.

Aside from stashing all your shorts at the back of your closet, what can you do about this infernal condition? Plenty, doctors say. To minimize their appearance:

• Get daily exercise. A 20- to 30-minute walk daily can keep the blood flowing.

• Don't gain too much weight.

• Avoid long periods of standing or sitting, and don't cross your legs when you sit.

• Elevate your legs whenever you get the chance to sit. When you're lying down, place a pillow under your feet.

• Avoid tight clothing, which can further restrict blood flow.

• Try wearing support hose, which are available in most maternity stores or pharmacies. Put them on before you get out of bed in the morning, before the blood has a chance to back up in your legs.

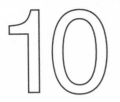

Getting Stronger

If it hadn't dawned on you before, you're probably starting to realize why it's important for your muscles to be strong now. This pregnancy stuff is physically demanding! If you've been doing our first trimester strength-training work, your legs should be more powerful already, which will help support the additional weight of your upper body in the coming months. Now it's time to bring your upper body, the bane of many women's strength-training programs, into the regimen. The moves we've included here probably aren't intense enough to give you a muscled look. But they will make you feel stronger and tougher and provide a mental edge that will be reassuring as you inch closer to labor day. In addition, strong arms will make lifting easier, especially as your abs get weaker and your belly becomes more cumbersome, and a strong back will help pull your shoulders and spine into alignment by offsetting the downward drag of your breasts and belly.

Most of the following exercises can be done standing or sitting in a chair. If you're comfortable standing you can continue to do so, but watch carefully for any signs of light-headedness. The American College of Obstetricians and Gynecologists recommends that you avoid long periods of motionless standing, which can cause blood to pool in your legs. We haven't included any exercises in the supine position, since an estimated 10 percent of pregnant women have low blood pressure, light-headedness, and even nausea when they lie on their backs—the result of the growing uterus compressing the vena cava, a large vein that returns blood to the heart.

How to Cope with Constipation and Hemorrhoids

Just when you've put your nausea and fatigue behind you, you've got two more problems, and these are also behind you—literally. Glamorous this isn't, but beginning sometime in the second trimester, constipation and hemorrhoids are a fact of life for many pregnant women.

Here's why: Between weeks 14 and 28, your uterus balloons to accommodate your growing baby. There's only so much room at the inn, however. As your womb expands, it starts crowding the other contents of your gut, namely your stomach and intestines, which are already on the sluggish side, thanks to the progesterone that's working to keep muscle contractions at bay. The result is a system that's stopped up as surely as if you'd put a cork in it. To help things flow a little easier, make sure you get plenty of fiber from fruits, vegetables, and whole grains; drink at least eight, and preferably ten, 8-ounce glasses of water daily; and try to fit in some exercise every day. A half-hour walk is particularly helpful. Still stopped up? Ask your doctor if she can recommend a stool softener that's safe to use during pregnancy.

In the meantime, don't be surprised if you start finding small painful lumps in your rectal area. In a classic case of Mother Nature adding insult to injury, hard-to-pass bowel movements often result in hemorrhoids (also known as piles because of their resemblance to a pile of grapes), or swollen veins in your rectum. Hemorrhoids can be supremely uncomfortable, causing itching and bleeding, but they won't do any permanent damage, except maybe to your vanity. Fortunately, most cases of hemorrhoids respond well to home treatment. Here's what to do:
• Treat your constipation. Curing the cause is half the battle.
• Do Kegel exercises. These classic pregnancy exercises, in which you contract the muscles of your pelvic floor, are beneficial because they improve circulation to the general area. (See our exercise chapters for several versions of this simple exercise.)
• Take a soothing sitz bath daily. Most drugstores carry the special shallow sitz bath tubs that fit over your toilet.
• Avoid standing or sitting for long stretches. Both can put extra pressure on your bottom, which only exacerbates the problem. Instead, try to lie down on your side as much as possible. (Lying on your back increases the pressure in your rectum as well.)
• Apply ice packs or soak the area in witch hazel. These treatments may not cure the problem, but they can provide some relief from the symptoms.
• Avoid inflatable hemorrhoid pillows. Shaped like rings or doughnuts, they may make you feel better temporarily, but they can actually backfire, making the problem worse by increasing the pressure on your anus.

LATERAL RAISE

Muscles it targets: Lateral deltoid.

Why do it: To help with everyday lifting and carrying motions and to create a strong, attractive curve in your shoulder—a sort of natural shoulder pad.

How to do it correctly: Sit on the edge of a chair with your feet flat on the floor a comfortable distance apart. With your spine straight and your abs pulled in firmly, hold a weight in each hand, arms by your sides, palms facing inward. Slowly raise the weights out to your sides to shoulder height, keeping your palms facing downward. Don't rotate your arms or lock your elbows. Hold for a count of two, then slowly lower the weights to the starting position. Exhale as you lift; inhale as you lower. Repeat 8 to 12 times. Work your way up to three sets.

Things to bear in mind: Keep your neck relaxed. As you raise your arms, pull your shoulders down. If you experience shoulder pain, lift the weights only as high as is comfortable.

To make this move slightly harder: Use heavier weights.

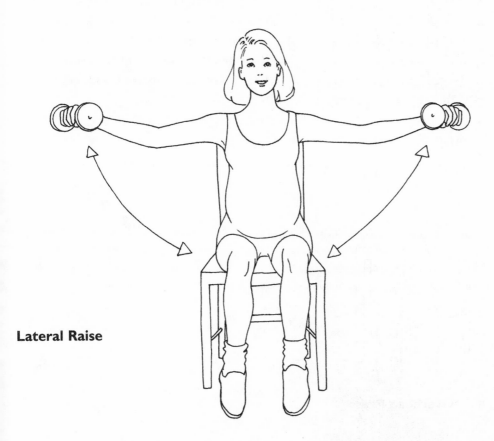

Lateral Raise

OVERHEAD PRESS

Muscles it targets: Deltoids.

Why do it: To create balance in your upper body muscles and shape your shoulders.

How to do it correctly: Sit on the edge of a chair with your feet flat on the floor a comfortable distance apart. With your spine straight and your abs pulled in firmly, hold a weight in each hand with palms facing down, bend your elbows in front of you so that your forearms are parallel and the weights are lifted to neck height with palms facing outward. This is your starting position. Keeping your arms parallel through the motion, push the weights up overhead without locking your elbows. Then lower the weights to the starting position. Exhale as you lift; inhale as you lower. Repeat 8 to 12 times. Work your way up to three sets.

Things to bear in mind: Your back will want to arch—don't let it. If you feel you need more support, place pillows behind your back or sit against the seat back. Keep the weights directly over your shoulders. Moving them out of alignment could put your shoulder tendon in jeopardy.

To make this move slightly harder: Use heavier weights. Lift and lower slowly.

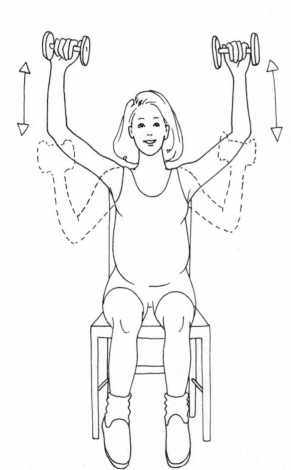

Overhead Press

TRICEPS EXTENSION

Muscles it targets: Triceps.

Why do it: To stave off jiggly "grandma" arms and give you more strength to push things—vacuums, strollers, swings.

How to do it correctly: Sit on the edge of a chair with your feet flat on the floor a comfortable distance apart. With your spine straight and your abs pulled in firmly, hold a weight in each hand directly over your head as high as you can without locking your elbows. Your palms should be facing each other, and your knuckles should be pressed together. Keeping your arms alongside your ears, bend your elbows and slowly lower the weights toward the backs of your shoulders. Keep your hands together. Lower the weights as far as you can without arching your back or moving your head. Hold for a count of two. Slowly return to the starting position. Exhale as you lower; inhale as you lift. Repeat 8 to 12 times. Work your way up to three sets.

Things to bear in mind: Keep your spine straight and your chin level. If you find that you're arching your back, use lighter weights.

To make this move slightly harder: Use heavier weights.

INTERNAL AND EXTERNAL ROTATORS

Muscles it targets: The four small muscles of the rotator cuff in your shoulder.

Why do it: You use these small, somewhat delicate muscles almost every time you move your arms. They're especially important when you swim the freestyle stroke and serve a tennis ball.

How to do it correctly: Sit on the edge of a chair with your feet flat on the floor a comfortable distance apart. With your spine straight and your abs pulled in firmly, hold a weight in your right hand, letting your left arm hang at your side. Keeping your right elbow tucked close to your body, bend your elbow, lifting the weight in front of you until your elbow forms a right angle. Holding the upper part of your right arm steady, slowly exhale and rotate the lower part of your right arm to the left until it touches your belly. Slowly inhale and rotate the arm back to center. Repeat 8 to 12 times. Then, starting with your right arm in the center position, rotate the lower part of the arm as far as you can to the right. Slowly rotate the arm back to center. Repeat 8 to 12 times. Work your way up to three sets. Repeat on the left side.

Things to bear in mind: Use light weights. These muscles are prone to injury. Don't bend your wrist.

To make this move slightly harder: Use heavier weights, but err on the side of caution so you don't overwork these muscles.

UPPER BACK CRUNCH

Muscles it targets: Erector spinae, lats, and traps.

Why do it: It will help you get in touch with the muscles of your upper back, which in turn can create greater postural awareness. It can also relieve upper back pain caused by your growing breasts and belly.

How to do it correctly: Sit on the edge of a chair with your feet flat on the floor a comfortable distance apart. With your spine straight and your abs pulled in firmly, extend your arms out to your sides at shoulder height, your palms facing backward. Pulse your arms behind you slowly and gently, as if you were trying to squeeze your shoulder blades together. Repeat 8 to 12 times. Work your way up to three sets.

Things to bear in mind: This move is effective only if you concentrate on squeezing your back muscles as you work.

To make this move slightly harder: Hold light weights in your hands.

KNEE LIFT

Muscles it targets: Transverse, rectus abdominis, and hip flexors (muscles that lie at the front of your hips).

Why do it: To maintain a strong center, which will help prevent lower back pain, to give you more strength for pushing the baby out, and to help you get your body back more quickly after delivery.

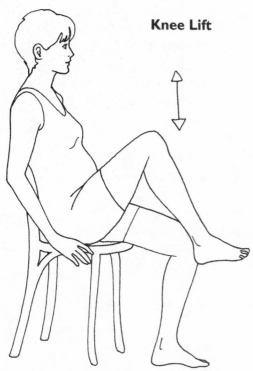

Knee Lift

How to do it correctly: Sit on the edge of a chair with your feet flat on the floor a comfortable distance apart. Place your hands, palms down, under your rear end. Pull in your abdominals and tilt your pelvis slightly under. Then pull your left knee to your chest. Hold for a count of one. Then contract your abs even further as you lower your left foot to the floor. Return your pelvis to a neutral position. Repeat 8 to 12 times. Then switch to the right leg. Work your way up to three sets.

Things to bear in mind: Unless you concentrate on pulling in your abdominals, your hip flexors will do all the work.

To make this move slightly harder: Wear light ankle weights.

SEATED CRUNCH

Muscles it targets: Transverse and rectus abdominis.

Why do it: To strengthen the muscles that will help you during labor.

How to do it correctly: Sit on the edge of a chair with your feet flat on the floor a comfortable distance apart. Place your hands around your belly as if you were hugging the baby. Exhale as you pull in your abdominals slowly to a count of five. Inhale as you release them slowly to a count of five. Repeat 8 to 12 times. Work your way up to three sets.

Things to bear in mind: Imagine you're trying to pull your belly button in toward your spine. Work slowly, concentrating on the contraction in your abdominals.

To make this move slightly harder: Once you've pulled your abdominals in as far as they will go, hold for a count of two. Then slowly release.

HAMSTRING AND GLUTE CURL (see chapter 6, page 69)

DUCK SQUAT (see chapter 6, page 71)

INTERMEDIATE KEGEL

Muscles it targets: Pubococcygeus, or PC muscle (see page 16)

Why do it: A strong pelvic floor is also a supple pelvic floor, which means it will stretch more easily when it comes time to push your baby out.

How to do it correctly: Sit on a chair or on the floor with your back against a wall, your legs slightly spread. Tighten the PC muscle and hold for 10 seconds. Do 8 to 12 reps. Work your way up to three sets.

Things to bear in mind: You may feel the contraction fade during the 10 seconds. If you do, just reassert the contraction.

To make this move slightly harder: Do it while in the duck squat position.

Plié with Leg Lift

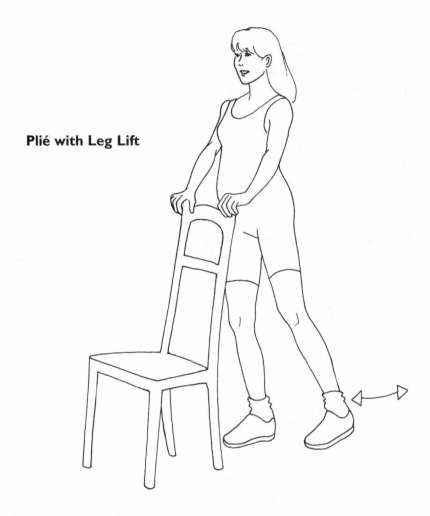

PLIÉ WITH LEG LIFT

Muscles it targets: Quadriceps, hamstrings, glutes, and outer thigh muscles.

Why do it: To build on the leg strength you've achieved with the plié alone.

How to do it correctly: Stand with your feet slightly wider than hip-distance apart with your toes turned out gently (to whatever degree feels comfortable), your knees slightly bent, and your abs pulled in firmly. Tuck your butt under slightly to prevent your back from arching. Holding on to a chair for support, bend your knees as far as you can while keeping your spine straight. Straighten your legs and lift your right leg up and out to the side. Keep your foot flexed. Lower the leg and immediately repeat the plié, this time lifting the left leg when you come up. Repeat 8 to 12 times. (Note: One full move includes two pliés, plus one right leg lift and one left leg lift.) Work your way up to three sets.

Things to bear in mind: To get the full benefit of this move, work slowly but maintain constant motion.

To make this move slightly harder: Wear light ankle weights.

POSTURE PRESS

Muscles it targets: Erector spinae, lats, and traps.

Why do it: To counteract the tendency to slouch and to prevent lower back pain.

How to do it correctly: Stand against a wall with your knees relaxed and your feet about hip-width apart, about 12 inches from the wall. Pull your stomach muscles in toward the wall, exhale, and press your head, shoulders, upper back, and hips into the wall. Then, keeping your spine straight and your muscles taut, push your upper body away from the wall with your hands. Repeat several times daily.

Things to bear in mind: This move puts your body in the proper position for your everyday life.

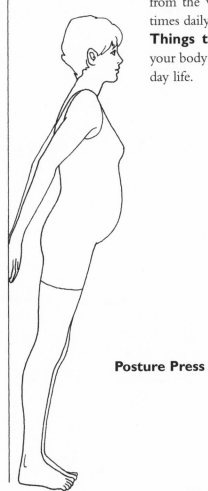

Posture Press

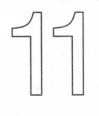

Enhancing Flexibility

We hope stretching has become second nature by now, and that you do it almost unconsciously as you're going about your daily tasks. If so, you're probably standing a bit taller and feeling more comfortable inside your changing body. Bravo! That means your workouts are, well, working out. If not, it's time to reconfirm that commitment. Skimp on stretching now, and you'll pay the price soon, with lower back pain, calf cramps, poor posture, and any number of other random problems.

Scary suggestions aside, stretching can go a long way toward keeping you centered, both physically and emotionally, especially now that your body is in full morph mode. Think of flexibility as the Zen element of exercise, the component that soothes both mind and body by giving you the opportunity to slow down and take stock. Are you holding tension in your neck and jaw? Is your posture beginning to deteriorate? Do your hamstrings feel tight? Are you stressed out? Overworked? Anxious? Fearful about what's still to come?

Use your 30-second stretching breaks throughout the day to let go of the physical and mental tension that can keep you from enjoying (or at least acknowledging) how miraculous this whole pregnancy thing is. Breathing deeply throughout the stretches can enhance their effectiveness as well as clear your mind and slough off stress. Try to be mentally present as you stretch to get the most out of each move. If your body feels inflexible and awkward, work within your limitations. This isn't about increasing your flexibility so much as maintaining it and giving your body the opportunity to adjust to its new conditions. Remember: Stretching isn't a competitive event. Extend only as far as is comfortable, then allow your body to relax into that position.

Since we outlined a safe, effective full-body flexibility routine in chapter 7, we recommend you continue that program throughout pregnancy. Here, we offer some additional suggestions specifically designed to combat problems that can crop up in the second trimester, such as poor posture and lower back discomfort. Add these to your daily routine to keep your body in proper working order. Before you try these new moves, take a minute to review the basic rules of stretching outlined in chapter 7 (pages 76–77).

HEAD CIRCLES

Muscles it targets: Neck and upper back.

Why do it: To release tension in your neck and shoulders and enhance postural awareness.

How to do it correctly: Sitting in a comfortable position, slowly drop your chin to your chest, then roll your head to the right, to the back, to the left, and around to the front. If there is a spot that's particularly tight, stop and allow that area to stretch a bit more.

When to do it: When you're sitting at your desk, watching television, taking a shower.

SPINE AND UPPER LEG STRETCH

Muscles it targets: Hamstrings, lower back, lats.

Why do it: To lengthen and relax your spine, to release the tension in the backs of your legs, and to ease shoulder tension.

How to do it correctly: Stand several feet in front of a table, chairback, or countertop. Bending at the hips, lower your upper body so it's parallel to the floor. With your arms outstretched, place your palms on the surface in front of you. Feel your weight sinking through your heels and the gentle release of your back muscles. Don't lock your knees or arch or round your back. If the stretch is uncomfortable, adjust your position slightly by taking a small step forward and moving your hands farther apart. Hold the stretch. To release it, bend your knees and roll up slowly, vertebra by vertebra.

When to do it: After sitting for long periods, after walking, before bed.

TRICEPS STRETCH

Muscles it targets: Triceps and shoulder.

Why do it: To open up your shoulders and keep your arms loose.

How to do it correctly: Reach your right hand overhead and behind you as if you were trying to scratch your upper back. With your right elbow pointed toward the ceiling, hold on to it with your left hand, pulling gently until you feel an easy stretch. Hold the stretch. Repeat with the left arm.

When to do it: When you're sitting at your desk, after you've been driving, when you're in the shower.

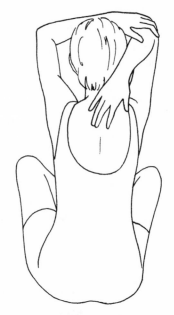

Triceps Stretch

CHEST OPENER

Muscles it targets: Pecs and delts.

Why do it: To improve your posture.

How to do it correctly: Lace your fingers behind your head, with your elbows pointing straight out to the sides. Gently pull your shoulder blades together. Hold the stretch for 10 seconds, then release. Repeat three times.

When to do it: When you're sitting at your desk, eating breakfast, watching TV.

SHOULDER STRETCH

Muscles it targets: Delts, pecs, and upper back.

Why do it: To reduce upper back hunching.

How to do it correctly: Reach your left hand, palm outward, behind your back, as close to the center of your shoulder blades as you can manage, with your elbow pointing toward the floor. Then reach your right arm overhead with your elbow pointing toward the ceiling, and try to link fingers with your left hand. If you can't, try to touch your fingertips as you exhale. Hold the stretch. Repeat on the other side.

When to do it: After you've been driving or sitting on a bus, when you're at your desk, after a walk.

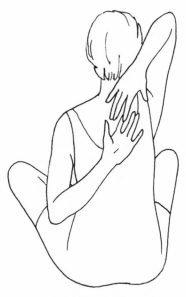

Shoulder Stretch

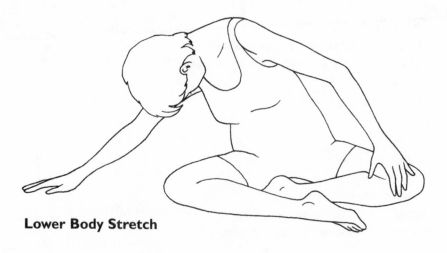

Lower Body Stretch

LOWER BODY STRETCH

Muscles it targets: Hip, thigh, and lower back.

Why do it: To open up your pelvis and lengthen muscles in your lower back.

How to do it correctly: Sit cross-legged with the toes of your left foot lying in the crease of your bent right knee. Place your right hand on your right knee and press down gently. Then lower your chin to your chest, rotate your torso to the left, and drop your chest toward your left leg, allowing your belly to drop to the inside of the leg. Keep your left hand on the floor for support. Drop your torso only as far as you can without rounding your spine. Hold the stretch. Repeat on the other side.

When to do it: After you exercise, when you're watching TV, before you go to bed.

How to Cope with Low Back Pain

Even if you're fortunate enough to avoid most of the annoying aches and ailments of pregnancy, chances are you'll experience at least a minor brush with back pain. Why? Because a number of pregnancy-related factors conspire to give you an achy back.

For one thing, as your belly grows your center of gravity shifts forward, causing your lower back to arch. This position places undue stress on the muscles in the area, which are forced to work overtime to correct the out-of-whack weight distribution. If you went into pregnancy with washboard abs, the chances your back will withstand the pressure are greater. But for most of us, who were slightly squishy in the middle to begin with, the pregnancy-induced postural changes send our backs straight into distress.

A collaborator in the back-pain conspiracy is diastasis, a condition in which the two halves of your abdominal muscles separate, which causes them to be weaker still. The weaker your abs, the harder your back has to work to keep your body upright.

Want more bad news? Back pain tends to get worse as your belly gets bigger. That's why it's important to take the appropriate steps sooner rather than later to combat this pervasive ailment:

• Keep weight gain in check. Extra pounds only place added stress on your already overburdened back.

• Commit to ab work. It's never too late to start gaining abdominal strength. See chapter 10 for exercises that are safe now.

• Stash the stilettos (or even high pumps) until after the baby is born. High heels tend to accentuate the curve in your lower back.

• Sit properly. Sitting places an incredible strain on your back, especially when you do it on backless stools or benches that offer nothing in the way of support. Seek out straight-back chairs with firm seats, and when you're sitting, don't cross your legs; do elevate them slightly (a few books or a low stool will give them enough lift to take the strain off your back).

• Practice perfect posture. Tuck your butt slightly under to tip your pelvis back into position and decrease the curve in your lower back; bring your head back into alignment with your body (imagine a string pulling the top of your head up toward the sky) and prevent your shoulders from sinking into the lazy woman's slouch.

• Lift carefully. See page 93 for a description of proper lifting technique.

• Avoid long periods of standing.

• Soothe yourself with heat. A heating pad wrapped in a towel or a warm bath can provide some relief for an aching back.

THE
third trimester

Your Changing Body

Cardiovascular Fitness

Getting Stronger

Enhancing Flexibility

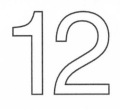

12 Your Changing Body

You're in the home stretch! When you look in the mirror it may seem hard to believe that a mere six months ago your baby weighed only a few ounces and you were still wearing clothes that, from where you stand now, look like they'd fit a Barbie doll. What may be even harder to believe, especially if your skin already feels like it's stretched across your abdomen like Saran Wrap, is that now is when the baby's *real* weight gain begins. In fact, over the next few months, your snug little bug is going to start getting a lot more snug as he or she doubles or even triples in size.

As your baby grows you're going to grow, too, in a way you've never grown before—out. Get ready to have girth, girl, because sooner or later (probably sooner) you're going to feel like a medicine ball with legs, a condition giving new meaning to everyday activities like getting out of bed and tying your shoes, much less working out. And you thought labor began when your contractions started. Ha! If carrying around an extra 20 to 35 (or more) pounds isn't laborious, we don't know what is! So give yourself a big pat on the back (or any special treat that fits your budget, from lipstick to diamond earrings), because you're doing the kind of work every minute of every day that would make the buffest gym rat grunt and groan.

Since you're getting a fair amount of exercise every time you move, your workout routine will understandably undergo some modifications in the next few months. But that doesn't mean you should hang up your sneakers and extralarge sweatpants for the duration of gestation. As long as you have your doctor's consent, staying active now is important for your health and well-being, and it will have fairly immediate rewards: You'll be strong for your impending labor, and your body will bounce back faster once you're a full-fledged babe-in-arms mother.

What's changing now? Just about everything, but here are the biggies—the things that will put extra work in every workout.

Posture and gait changes We described the round-shouldered, swaybacked posture typical during pregnancy in chapter 8, but now that your body is in full bloom, the tendency to look like a human S is even more pronounced. The more your belly pulls you forward, the more your lower back will hollow out and the more likely you are to suffer from lower back pain, especially if you spend lots of time on your feet. As a result, it's time to straighten up. Do our posture check in chapter 8, and adjust yourself accordingly.

Meanwhile, the heavier your belly gets and the more your hip joints loosen, the more your stride will be affected. In an effort to stabilize your off-kilter body, you may unconsciously start walking like a duck, with your feet splayed out to the sides. Once your baby's head descends into the birth canal, which usually happens in first pregnancies about two to four weeks before delivery, the waddle effect will become even more conspicuous. Likewise, the larger you get the more your stride will shorten, both when you walk and when you run, and jogging may start looking more like shuffling since you won't be able to pick your feet up as high as you normally did.

Awareness is the key to taking these gait changes in stride. If you allow your body to move in ways that feel comfortable, slow your pace accordingly, focus on keeping your footfalls as light and graceful as possible, avoid activities requiring rapid changes in direction, and keep a wary eye out for potential tripping hazards, you should be able to remain injury-free for the rest of your pregnancy.

Shortness of breath Even if you could run 6-minute miles in your prepregnancy life, you may find yourself huffing and puffing at the top of a flight of stairs once you're in your last trimester. For superfit women, this can be the most bitter blow of all. Rest assured, this isn't happening because you've suddenly lost every ounce of physical fitness you've worked so hard to attain. It's simply the result of overcrowded conditions inside your body.

By the time you're 36 weeks pregnant, your uterus has expanded to about 1,000 times its usual size. Not surprisingly, the more it grows the more it presses against your diaphragm, the muscle that separates your abdominal and chest cavities. This gives your lungs less room in which to operate. (It also restricts other organs, including your stomach, making symptoms like heartburn and indigestion more likely. See "How to Cope with Heartburn" (opposite). Once the baby drops into the birth canal, you should get some relief. In the meantime, maintaining good posture can open up your chest and at least partially liberate your lungs.

Nobody likes to feels winded, but it can be especially troubling now, so much so that you may be tempted to take this symptom as a sign that it's time to quit exercising. Not so, say researchers in the field, who have found evidence quite to the contrary. A study published in 1998 in the American College of Sports Medicine's journal *Medicine and Science in Sports and Exercise* compared the breathing rates of sedentary pregnant women with those of pregnant women who rode a stationary bike three days a week for 25 minutes per session. Researchers found the pregnant exercisers had less severe symptoms of breathlessness, which led them to speculate that physical conditioning may make the mechanics of breathing more efficient and, as a result, may actually help prevent and treat pregnancy-induced shortness of breath. The bottom line: If you feel out of breath, slow down, but by all means stay as active as you can because of the potential benefit.

Increased heart rate We mentioned in chapter 1 that during the first trimester your heart rate increases as a result of all the extra blood a pregnant body requires. Since then, your resting pulse has gradually sped up even more, so that during this trimester it's at least 15 beats per minute above what it was in your prepregnancy state. This shift, combined with

How to Cope with Heartburn

That pizza looked mighty appealing when it was sitting on your plate, but now that it's hit your stomach it's paying a repeat visit in the unpleasant form of gastric reflux, aka heartburn.

Pregnancy hormones can make heartburn more likely practically from the moment of conception, but once your uterus has successfully crowded your stomach and other internal organs into whatever nook or cranny they can find in your abdominal cavity, this symptom becomes even more pronounced. The best defense is to replace your three squares with lots of small, low-fat meals and frequent snacks. This style of eating doesn't overload your stomach, a condition that results in the backing up of stomach acids into your esophagus. Eating slowly, chewing each bite thoroughly, avoiding food within several hours of bedtime, and sleeping with your head elevated at least 6 inches will also help.

Another trick: Chew a stick of gum after you eat. A study from the University of Alabama found that pregnant women who chewed an average of 4.5 sticks of gum per day suffered heartburn less often and with less intensity than when they didn't chew gum. If the problem is severe, ask your doctor if you can take one of the over-the-counter antacids or H_2 blockers.

your body's increased oxygen requirements due to your increased weight, means there will be an unmistakable decline in your ability to maintain a given exercise intensity. Don't take this as a sign of failure. Your body is working just as hard to exercise at a slower pace, and any prolonged physical activity at all will help maintain your cardiovascular fitness.

Weight gain Until the last month of pregnancy you should aim to gain about a pound a week, but fear not. Most of this won't end up on your hips and thighs. Your baby is fattening up for survival outside the womb, so at least half of this extra weight will be carried by your wee one. Still, every extra ounce may be distressing to you as you watch your belly inflate as surely as if it were a helium-filled balloon. Trust us, you won't pop, much as it might feel like you're going to. But that overstuffed feeling may serve to curb your appetite as you head into these final months. Try to eat more small meals and redouble your efforts to make every calorie a healthy one.

The extra weight will also have an impact on your energy and your motivation to exercise. Don't force yourself if you truly don't feel up to it, but if you're in that waffling mode—weighing the appeal of a nice walk against the temptation of a bowl of ice cream, say—try to summon your inner resources to get out the door (and avoid the freezer as you go). If you do, you'll probably find that physical activity will revitalize both body and soul, giving your spirits at least as much of a boost as a scoop of Häagen-Dazs without the physical repercussions.

By the end of this trimester, you should be tipping the scales somewhere between 25 and 35 pounds above your normal weight. Where does all that extra weight go? Here's the average breakdown, according to the American College of Obstetricians and Gynecologists:

Pregnancy Weight Distribution

Maternal stores (fat, protein, and other nutrients)	7 pounds
Increased fluid	4 pounds
Increased blood	4 pounds
Breast growth	2 pounds
Uterus	2 pounds
Baby (average weight)	7.5 pounds
Amniotic fluid	2 pounds
Placenta	1.5 pounds

How to Cope with Carpal Tunnel Syndrome

The tingling, swelling, and pain in the wrists, hands, and arms characterizing carpal tunnel syndrome are most commonly associated with long hours at a keyboard, but pregnant women often experience this distressing ailment even if they've never touched a computer. The cause is swelling in the carpal tunnel of the wrist, which compresses the nerves in the area.

Because fluids accumulate in your hands during the day, the symptoms of carpal tunnel syndrome often strike in the middle of the night. If you awaken to numb arms and hands night after night, it's a good bet you've succumbed to this pregnancy-related ailment. Fortunately, the symptoms usually subside once the baby is born. Until then, follow these wrist-saving tips:

• Don't sleep on your hands.
• Try to sleep with your wrists in a neutral position, either flat on the bed or splinted to hold them straight.
• Soak your hands in ice water to reduce the swelling.
• When numbness and tingling strike, hold your hand down and shake it gently.
• Stretch it out: Hold your left arm out in front of you from the shoulder with your palm facing away from your body, fingers pointed down. With your right hand, gently press your left hand toward you for ten counts. Then, do the same thing with your fingers pointing up. Do three repetitions. Repeat with the right hand.
• Make sure you keep wrists in a neutral position when lifting weights or exercising with bands or tubing.
• If the problem is severe, ask your doctor about cortisone injections.

Your Pregnant Brain

Wondering why your IQ seems to have dropped a point for every pound you've gained? Why you've discovered the tinfoil in the freezer and the ice cream dripping all over the pantry? Why some pesky poltergeist keeps hiding your car keys, your glasses, the book you were reading? Forgetfulness, spaciness, and an inability to concentrate go with the territory of pregnancy, and many doctors now believe they may have a very real biological cause. According to the results of several studies, a mother-to-be's brain actually shrinks late in pregnancy. Although there's no proof this is the cause of the annoying brain-drain syndrome striking most pregnant women, it's an intriguing possibility.

Helping Hands: Massage Tips for Partners

Your back hurts. Your abdomen aches. Your shoulders are tired and your neck feels cramped. Sure, you could take a bath or curl up on the couch. But isn't it time your partner got into the act? He can provide a little sensual healing in the form of a soothing massage.

Massage not only helps work the physical kinks from your hardworking body but also provides emotional comfort, easing the fear and anxiety that often niggles at you by day (and totally grips you by night). It's also a great way to reconnect with your partner, who may feel left out of the pregnancy experience and somewhat sexually neglected, if, like many women in the third trimester, you're finding it hard to work up much enthusiasm for sex.

Before you begin, get your doctor's okay, because you shouldn't have a massage if you have certain conditions such as varicose veins. To set the scene, make sure the room is comfortably warm. Enhance the mood by dimming the lights and playing soft music. Pull a chair up to a table-top and place some cushy pillows on the table. Then sit down in the chair and lay your head and shoulders on the pillows, leaving your back exposed for the therapeutic massage. Now, give this book to your man. It's time to let the dad-to-be try his hand at nurturing.

For Husbands or Helpmates

1. Place your palms on her lower back and, while exerting gentle pressure, move your hands up her back on either side of her spine. When you get to her neck, move your hands out toward her shoulders, then back down along the outer edges of her back to the starting point. Repeat this broad stroke several times, making your movements as seamless and fluid as possible.

2. Place your hands on her lower back with your thumbs together in the center, your fingers out toward the edges of her back. Working your thumbs in a circular motion, massage her pelvic bones. Move your hands slowly up the center of her lower back, then work your way out to the sides and over the hips and upper buttocks.

3. Place your thumbs on either side of her lower spine, and, working again in a gentle, circular motion, move them slowly toward the upper back. If you come across painful areas, have her take a deep breath and imagine she is sending the breath to the painful spot.

4. Once you reach the upper back, place your thumbs at the base of the neck and work in a circular motion as you move along the neck out toward the shoulders.

Experts do know the phenomenon isn't all in your head. A researcher at the University of Southern California tested nineteen highly educated pregnant women and found they all had a decreased ability to concentrate and retain information in their short-term memory as well as learn new information. So, if you feel a little intellectually challenged these days, it's because you are. No one knows precisely why this pregnancy-induced feeblemindedness occurs, but it's most likely due to a combination of things —raging hormones, inadequate sleep, maybe even a biological imperative telling you to turn your attention inward rather than outward.

Whatever the cause, we recommend you heed this inner directive by giving your brain a break and taking some time to dwell on, well, just being. As Sylvia Boorstein's meditation book urges: Don't just do something, sit there. Cut back your work hours, turn off the television, put away the vacuum, and enjoy a few well-deserved moments of peace, quiet, and solitude. You can spend this time daydreaming about the baby, practicing some of the relaxation techniques we provided in chapter 4, or simply floating in the ether of your absentmindedness.

A word of warning: What you may find once you slow down enough to let yourself think is that you're overcome by feelings of fear and anxiety about what lies ahead. If you haven't already been doing so, now is a good time to work on your breathing. Try this confidence-building exercise that will help slough off anxiety and get you emotionally in shape for labor: Sit in any position that's comfortable, close your eyes, and allow the muscles of your face, neck, and shoulders to relax. Place your hands lightly on your belly. As you inhale, feel your belly expand and imagine your breath carrying strength and energy to all your muscles and organs, particularly your uterus. As you exhale, visualize yourself expelling the fears, insecurities, and uncertainties that wake you up in the middle of the night. Do 8 to 12 breaths, then relax.

Fitness Q & A

I like to take a bath after I exercise, but I've heard that you're supposed to avoid bathing in the last month or so of pregnancy. Is that right?

No. Unless your water has broken, you can ignore this pregnancy "don't" along with the other ones warning you away from physical activity, sex, or spicy foods. In fact, right about now the warm water and peaceful atmosphere of a dimly lit bathroom might be just what the doctor ordered. Still, you'll need to exercise more caution than usual when you steal a few moments for a relaxing soak. For one thing, you should keep the water in the comfortably warm range instead of piping hot to make sure your baby doesn't get overheated. Secondly, you should place a bath mat or some other non-slip surface in the bottom of the tub since slips are more likely when you can't see your feet. Along the same lines, hold on to an immovable object or ask for your partner's assistance when you're entering and exiting the tub.

 My baby doesn't seem to move at all when I exercise. Should I be worried?

Probably not. The motion of your body has most likely lulled the little critter off to sleep. By the end of this trimester, your baby's movements will slow in general, mostly because there's less room in your uterus for him or her to perform baby gymnastics. Instead of the sweet, fluttery kicks of the second trimester, you're likely to feel painful jabs and dramatic rolls as your baby struggles to get comfortable in his or her cramped quarters. If you're truly worried about your baby's activity level, do a kick test. For several days in a row, lie down on your left side on the couch after you've eaten breakfast (or any meal). Count the number of movements you feel in 5 minutes so you can compare your baby's activity from day to day. If you feel fewer than 10 movements in an hour, call your doctor.

 My friends who have kids keep telling me that walking is a great way to trigger labor once you're close to your due date. Is that true?

Although women who are within a week or so of their due dates have been known to try everything from nipple stimulation, which promotes the release of the natural labor stimulant oxytocin, to sex, which delivers a shot of prostaglandin-saturated semen to your cervix and also may cause contractions, nothing you can do at home has been definitively proven to trigger labor, including walking. (In the hospital, health care providers promote labor by administering Pitocin, the synthetic cousin of oxytocin.) Once you're in labor, however, most obstetrical experts believe walking can keep things progressing, partly because the upright position allows gravity to work its magic.

The Truth About Labor

There's no sense in whitewashing reality: Labor hurts. A lot. Many women compare it to menstrual cramps in the beginning, but it usually (not always) advances to a level that can only be called excruciating. Fortunately, there are a couple of things distinguishing labor pain from other random aches, and they make it a whole lot easier to bear.

For one thing, labor pain is pain you can prepare for. That's at least partly why you picked up this book, why you've been exercising for the past six or so months, why you should take a childbirth preparation class and learn everything you can about what's to come, why you've cross-examined every friend, relative, waitress, and grocery clerk about her birth experience. Getting your mind around the idea is half the battle, because it will help you circumvent the fear-tension-pain cycle, in which you get tense because you're scared, which makes your pain feel worse, which makes you more scared, more tense, and so on.

Secondly, labor pain is pain with a purpose, and, perhaps more importantly, pain with an end. It doesn't go on indefinitely (we promise), and, once it's over, you get the most astonishing jaw-dropper of a door prize you'll ever hope to see: a baby.

How long will you have to endure the pain before you get the prize? That depends. The American College of Obstetricians and Gynecologists (ACOG) says the average first labor lasts 12 to 14 hours, and subsequent labors are usually shorter. However, a study conducted at the University of New Mexico in Albuquerque, which looked at the labors of 1,500 healthy women, found that the first stage (during which the cervix dilates completely to 10 centimeters) of first labors lasts up to 19.4 hours; and mothers who had given birth before had a shorter first stage, up to 13.7 hours, not including the pushing stage, which can add up to 2 or more hours.

Keeping in mind that there's no such thing as a textbook labor, here's a typical labor profile, according to the ACOG:

The **first stage,** during which your cervix dilates, has three phases: early, active, and transition. During the **early phase,** you dilate to 5 centimeters. Mild contractions begin 15 to 20 minutes apart and last 60 to 90 seconds. Contractions gradually become more regular, until they are less than 5 minutes apart. During the **active phase,** your cervix dilates from 5 to 8 centimeters. Meanwhile, your contractions get stronger, progress to 3 minutes apart, and last about 45 seconds. During the **transition phase,** your cervix dilates from 8 to 10 centimeters. Your contractions are about 2 to 3 minutes apart and last about 1 minute.

The **second stage** of labor, which can last 2 hours or more, is the pushing stage. Contractions may slow to 2 to 5 minutes apart and last 60 to 90 seconds, but they'll feel different. They're usually more regular with a more well-defined rest period in between.

The **third stage** begins after the baby is born and ends when the placenta comes out. It typically lasts anywhere from several minutes to 15 to 20 minutes. Contractions may continue but are much less painful.

All in all, you should count on being miserable for a day, maybe more. But think about it this way: What's one day of agony compared with the years of pleasure (okay, and some agony, too) you'll derive from having a child?

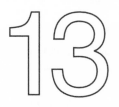

13 Cardiovascular Fitness

The extra weight you're now carrying is going to start weighing on you, literally, and that boundless energy you had during the second trimester will begin evaporating as surely as hot breath on a cold window. There are going to be more days when the idea of shuffling around the block, much less power walking, swimming, or bicycling, will make you feel like crawling into bed and pulling the covers up over your head. Go ahead and give in to the urge to slack off a little. But make a pact with yourself to get out the door at least three times a week, even if it's just for a 10-minute stroll.

Even minor bouts of activity will help keep your heart in shape and give you the endurance you'll need to get through the big event drawing ever closer. Moreover, staying somewhat active will help you keep some of the more onerous pregnancy villains—constipation, varicose veins, breathlessness, swelling, and fatigue—at bay.

Just to refresh your memory, we'd like you to take a peek at "The Seven Commandments of Pregnancy Fitness" listed on page 52. Now that you're good and pregnant, you should follow those rules as if they *were* sent down from on high. Likewise, you'll need to be more careful than ever before, because someday soon a new factor is going to complicate even the simplest activities—you won't be able to see your feet. That means, of course, you won't be able to see the ground beneath your feet, either, making stumbles, missteps, and falls more likely. As a result, you'll need to shake off that last-trimester fog as much as possible when you exercise so you can move with greater awareness and care.

In addition, if you've been playing sports requiring sudden moves and a good sense of balance, such as tennis or basketball, you may want to reconsider your choice of activities. True, if you were to fall on your belly, chances are your baby would be okay, because she or he is well protected by a buffer zone of fat and amniotic fluid. Still, do you really want that kind of concern on your conscience? For your own peace of mind, if nothing else, we believe it's wise to switch to walking, biking, or swimming until your body returns to some semblance of its former self.

As you exercise, you may start feeling a tightening in your abdomen. This is called a Braxton-Hicks contraction, a sort of labor warm-up often beginning sometime after the twentieth week of pregnancy and becoming more frequent in the last month. Unless these contractions are painful, predictable, and rhythmic, they're not real labor. But they are your cue to give your body a chance to rest. If you have Braxton-Hicks contractions as you're exercising, stop and focus on slow, deep breathing. Once they subside, you can continue at a slow pace, but stay in touch with your body and heed its signals.

You also need to watch for signs of pregnancy-induced high blood pressure, or preeclampsia, which occurs in about 7 percent of pregnancies and is more common in first-time mothers-to-be. Although it's typical for blood pressure to rise somewhat late in pregnancy, when it's accompanied by certain other changes it can signal the onset of preeclampsia. If an increase in blood pressure is accompanied by sudden weight gain—more than 2 pounds in a week, say—severe swelling, particularly of your hands and face, and protein in your urine (your doctor checks for this at every visit), you may need to be monitored closely and take it easy for the remaining duration of your pregnancy.

As you near your due date you may feel more like a Mack truck than a Porsche, but you need to realize your body is humming along like a fine-tuned machine. Even if you aren't as sprightly or as quick as you once were, you're every bit as strong, powerful, and physically vigorous—maybe more so. Now would be a great time to admire your hardworking body for the near-miraculous instrument it is, respect its current limitations, and keep in mind that your present condition is temporary.

If your baby is overdue, you can continue exercising as long as you have your doctor's okay. A daily walk might even help you deal with the natural anxiety you're going to be feeling, but we don't recommend you go on marathon walks or do any extended bouts of exercise. Better to save your energy for the work still in store for you and enjoy some activities you won't have a chance to do for a while—have dinner out with your partner, catch a movie, curl up with a good book, give yourself a manicure. Your days (and nights) of leisure are numbered. You might as well make the most of them.

How to Cope with Insomnia

It's ironic: Everyone from your doctor to your mother-in-law is advising you to get more rest, but researchers who study women's sleep patterns say the last trimester of pregnancy is one of the most difficult times in a woman's life to get a decent night's sleep. Not only are you more likely to be plagued by sleep disruptions—leg cramps, backache, heartburn, fetal movements, abdominal discomfort, and increased urination—but also your sleep, when you actually get it, is generally of poorer quality than that of nonpregnant women.

Studies show the amount of slow-wave, or deep, restorative sleep decreases as pregnancy progresses, as does the amount of REM sleep, during which dreaming typically occurs. Meanwhile, the number of awakenings increases as pregnancy draws to a close. In fact, the proportion of time you spend in bed sleeping (as opposed to tossing and turning) actually begins to decrease in the second trimester and continues to decline in the third trimester.

What's a bleary-eyed mother-to-be to do? For one thing, you should get daily exercise, but not within three or four hours of bedtime, which can rev you up and make sleep even more elusive. The most sleep-friendly exercise time: late afternoon. In addition to making your body fatigued and more primed for sleep, exercise can help prevent a typical pregnancy sleep disturber: restless leg syndrome. This jittery affliction that makes you feel like you constantly need to move or stretch your legs also may be relieved with leg massage, ice packs, or a heating pad.

Other sleep-promoting behaviors:
- Maintain a regular sleep/wake schedule.
- Eat a balanced diet.
- Avoid heavy or spicy foods within two or three hours of bedtime.
- Have a glass of milk before bed, because it contains L-tryptophan, an amino acid that some experts believe helps induce sleep.
- Write down your worries on index cards and tell yourself you'll think about them in the morning instead of in the middle of the night.
- Practice muscle relaxation techniques. Try counting backward from 100, feeling your body, from your toes up, relax a bit more with each number.
- Assume a comfortable position. Try curling up on your left side with a pillow underneath your belly and another one between your legs. If your back is uncomfortable, have your partner place another pillow in the small of your back.
- Try visualization. Picture yourself lying in a peaceful meadow beside a gurgling stream or on a warm beach with small waves lapping the shore. Breathe deeply and try to hear the sound of the water (if this makes you feel like you have to pee, imagine you're listening to the wind instead).

Guidelines for New Exercisers

Now is not a good time to launch a full-scale exercise assault on your newly rounded form. If you sat around eating Mallomars and playing dominoes during the first two trimesters, however, you can get your body in motion now, as long as you have your doctor's permission. The key to making that transition safely: Take it slowly. Ease into exercise by taking a slow 5-minute walk every day for two weeks. Then, increase your time (but not your pace), by taking a 10-minute walk every day for a week. After that, you can follow the beginner's walking program we describe in chapter 5.

Guidelines for Intermediate and Advanced Exercisers

Maybe you've been following one of our specially designed aerobic programs, or perhaps you've been taking a class you love. In any case, if you're in a groove that feels comfortable to you, stick with it as long as you can. If you start feeling too worn out, modify your intensity or duration or both. Now more than ever it's important that you trust your body and pay attention to what it's telling you.

We still feel walking is one of the best options around, so if you're interested in a good walking workout, refer to chapter 9, where we provide details of a program that includes some interval training. Or check out the following two options, either of which will get you through these last few months in good shape.

Stationary cycling If you're looking for a change of pace, a recumbent stationary bike, in which you pedal straight out in front of you, offers a great third trimester cardiovascular workout. For one thing, it provides ample room for a protruding belly. In addition, it offers back support, which can be appealing for anyone who's having lower back pain. Recumbent bikes have a further advantage over traditional uprights: They target your glutes and hamstrings better, a plus for anyone who is starting to worry about the expanding acreage in her backyard.

Stationary bikes offer a variety of programs, so you can choose one you like or do a different one every time to keep it interesting. If you like to set the bike on manual and stay in charge of the intensity, try our program.

the program: Ride slowly for 5 minutes to warm up. Then ride for 10 minutes at an easy to moderate pace. For the next 12 minutes, alternate 1-minute periods of moderately fast cycling (not sprinting) with 3-minute periods of easy to moderate cycling. Cool down for 5 minutes by cycling slowly.

Swimming You may find the frog kick required during breaststroke is uncomfortable now, so your swimming may be limited to freestyle. That's why our swimming workout for the third trimester adds another gadget to your repertoire: rubber swim fins. (Don't use scuba fins, which are too long and stiff.) They're a great option now because they give you more power and help counteract the drag of your growing belly so you won't tire as quickly. Meanwhile, they help you develop leg and ankle strength, both of which will serve you in good stead during labor and beyond.

the program: Swim 5 to 10 minutes at an easy pace to warm up. Then swim 100 yards at a moderate pace. Rest 1 minute. (If you don't feel adequately recovered after our recommended rest periods, give yourself more time.) Swim 200 yards at a moderate pace. Rest 2 minutes. Swim 300 yards at a moderate pace. Rest 3 minutes. Swim 200 yards at an easy to moderate pace. Rest 2 minutes. Swim 100 yards at an easy pace to cool down.

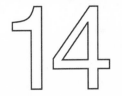

14 Getting Stronger

Strength training during the last trimester of pregnancy—when the mere act of getting out of bed takes on all the characteristics of a track-and-field event—can feel like a monumental challenge. Still, it's to your advantage to stick with the program. Modify your expectations, your exertion, even your effort, but hang in there. When you're pushing your baby out into the world or, later on, lifting her from her crib or zipping up your prepregnancy jeans, you'll be glad you did.

We've tried to make it as easy as possible for you to keep up your good work by creating a less intense version of the routines you've followed up to this point. As a result, most of the following moves can be done while you're sitting or lying down, the better to conserve energy even as you expend it. Even so, if you start feeling fatigued, take a breather. As your due date draws near, you might even want to break up your workout into several sessions during the day so you never overtax your body. There's nothing worse than going *into* labor feeling tired. Because of that, we've left out instructions for how to make the following moves more difficult. If you want more of a challenge, you can continue doing the workout from chapter 10, but the same precautions we mentioned then apply even more so now: Avoid long periods of motionless standing and don't exercise while lying flat on your back. Good luck. You're almost there.

SEATED POSTURE IMPROVER

Muscles it targets: Rhomboids, erector spinae, and traps.
Why do it: To keep your upper back strong, which will help you hold your head in alignment with your spine and reduce the risk of backaches.
How to do it correctly: Sit in a straight-back chair with your feet flat on the floor about hip-width apart and your abdominals pulled in firmly. Allow your arms to hang loosely by your sides. As you exhale, pull your shoulder

blades back toward the chair, feeling the muscles of your upper back contract. Hold for 3 seconds. (Breathe naturally. Don't hold your breath.) Inhale and release to the count of three. Repeat 8 to 12 times. If you're making each contraction count, there's no need to do more than one set.

Things to bear in mind: This movement is small and effective only if you concentrate on flexing the upper back muscles. As you squeeze your shoulder blades together, keep your shoulders and neck relaxed and your head erect.

DUCK SQUAT (see chapter 6, page 71)

BACK CURL

Muscles it targets: Strengthens abdominals; stretches lower back.

Why do it: To build power in your pushing muscles and ease lower back tension.

How to do it correctly: Position yourself on your hands and knees with your arms directly under your shoulders (elbows soft, not locked), your knees directly under your hips, your back straight, and your head in alignment with your spine. Inhale and feel your belly expand. As you exhale, pull your abs in toward your spine and round your back toward the ceiling, allowing your pelvis to tuck under. Hold for 3 seconds. (Breathe naturally. Don't hold your breath.) Inhale and return to the starting position. Repeat 8 to 12 times. If you're making each contraction count, there's no need to do more than one set.

Things to bear in mind: Keep your spine, neck, and face muscles relaxed, but don't allow your back to become concave when you return to the starting position.

SEATED ABDOMINAL CURL

Muscles it targets: Abdominals.

Why do it: To strengthen your midsection for the pushing stage of labor and simultaneously stretch your back.

How to do it correctly: Place several pillows on the floor. Sit in front of them with your spine straight, your knees bent, and your feet a comfortable distance from your butt. With your hands cupping the underside of your thighs for support, inhale and allow your lower back to collapse into the pillows by rounding your upper back forward and tucking your pelvis under. Then exhale and pull your abdominal muscles in toward your spine for 3 seconds. Inhale and return to the starting position. Repeat 8 to 12 times. If you're making each contraction count, there's no need to do more than one set.

Things to bear in mind: The movement is subtle, so focus on feeling the contraction in your abdominals. At the same time, feel your pubococcygeus (PC) muscle relaxing, a trick that mimics the actual physiological experience of pushing, when your abdominals will contract and your pelvic floor muscles will be opening up.

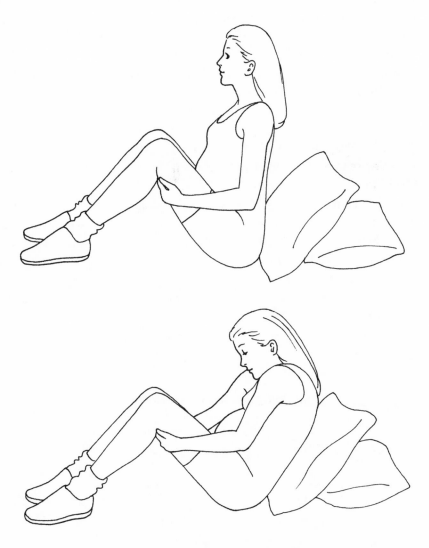

Seated Abdominal Curl

SIDE-LYING CRUNCH

Muscles it targets: Abdominals.

Why do it: To strengthen your abs for the pushing stage of labor.

How to do it correctly: Lie on your right side with your head resting comfortably on your right arm and your legs slightly bent. (To keep your neck in line with your spine, it may help to place a folded towel between your arm and head.) Place your left hand behind your neck and inhale. Then, lift your head slightly and exhale as you pull your left knee up toward your left elbow, feeling your abdominals contract as you execute the move. Inhale as you return to the starting position. Repeat 8 to 12 times. Turn onto your left side and repeat with your right leg. If you're making each contraction count, there's no need to do more than one set.

Things to bear in mind: Lift your head only slightly and allow it to relax on your lower arm between moves. Concentrate on working your abdominal muscles.

SIDE-LYING OUTER THIGH LIFT

Muscles it targets: Outer hip and thigh muscles (aka abductors).

Why do it: To provide extra support for your hardworking pelvic region.

How to do it correctly: Lie on your right side with your head resting comfortably on your right arm. (To keep your neck in line with your spine, it may help to place a folded towel between your arm and head.) Bend your knees so your thighs form a 45-degree angle with your hips. Planting your left hand on the floor in front of you for support, exhale as you lift your left leg to hip height. Inhale as you return the leg to the starting position. Repeat 8 to 12 times. Turn onto your left side and repeat with your right leg. If you feel up to it, work your way up to three sets.

Side-lying Outer Thigh Lift

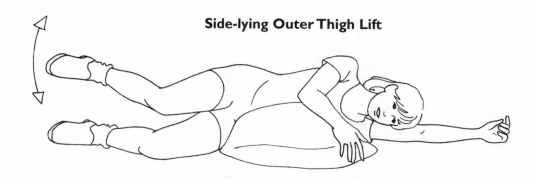

Things to bear in mind: Keep your abdominals contracted through the move, don't roll your hips forward or backward, and keep your leg in the same plane as you lift—don't allow the knee to point up or down.

SIDE-LYING INNER THIGH LIFT

Muscles it targets: Inner thigh muscles (aka adductors).

Why do it: To stave off the inner thigh jiggle that can occur after you gain and lose weight, and to help you perform better in a number of sports, including horseback riding, tennis, soccer, and dance.

How to do it correctly: Lie on your right side with your head resting comfortably on your right arm. (To keep your neck in line with your spine, it may help to place a folded towel between your arm and head.) Extend your right leg straight down. Bend your left knee and rest it in front of you on a pillow for support. Planting your left hand on the floor in front of you for support, exhale as you lift your right leg up as high as you can toward the ceiling, without rolling your hips forward or backward. Inhale as you lower the leg to the starting position. Repeat 8 to 12 times. Turn onto your left side and repeat with your left leg. If you feel up to it, work your way up to three sets.

Things to bear in mind: Keep the foot of your lifted leg flexed and your toes facing forward, not up or down. Keep your pelvis in a neutral position and your spine straight.

Side-lying Inner Thigh Lift

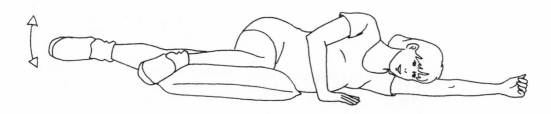

SIDE-LYING LATERAL RAISE

Muscles it targets: The lateral, or middle, of the deltoids.

Why do it: This muscle acts as a stabilizer when you lift, something you'll be doing more of shortly.

How to do it correctly: Lie on your right side with your head resting comfortably on your right arm. (To keep your neck in line with your spine, it may help to place a folded towel between your arm and head.) Bend your knees so your thighs form a 45-degree angle with your hips. Hold a light (2- to 5-pound) weight in your left hand. Keep your arm slightly bent and in line with your torso, palm down, the weight resting on your outer thigh. Exhale and slowly lift the weight to about 45 degrees. Inhale and lower it to the starting position. Repeat 8 to 12 times. Turn onto your left side and repeat with your right arm. If you feel up to it, work your way up to three sets.

Things to bear in mind: Keep your abs contracted throughout the move and your hips stacked. If you feel yourself rolling forward or backward, place a pillow under your tummy and behind you for support. As you lift, keep your wrist in a neutral position and the inside of your arm facing down to prevent shoulder rotation.

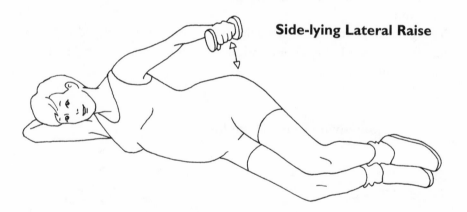

Side-lying Lateral Raise

SIDE-LYING BICEPS CURL

Muscles it targets: Biceps.

Why do it: To maintain arm strength for lifting and carrying your baby.

How to do it correctly: Lie on your right side with your head resting comfortably on your right arm. (To keep your neck in line with your spine, it may help to place a folded towel between your arm and head.) Bend your knees so your thighs form a 45-degree angle with your hips. Hold a light (2- to 5-pound) weight in your left hand; keep your palm facing toward the ceiling and the back of your hand resting on top of your outer thigh. Keeping your upper arm pressed against your side, exhale and slowly bend your elbow to 90 degrees. Inhale and slowly lower the weight to the starting position. Repeat 8 to 12 times. Turn onto your left side and repeat. If you feel up to it, work your way up to three sets.

Things to bear in mind: Keep your abs contracted throughout the move and your hips stacked. If you feel yourself rolling forward or backward, place a pillow under your tummy and behind you for support. As you lift, keep your wrist in a neutral position.

SIDE-LYING TRICEPS EXTENSION

Muscles it targets: Triceps.

Why do it: To prevent jiggly upper arms and keep your arms strong for lifting your baby.

How to do it correctly: Lie on your right side with your head resting comfortably on your right arm. (To keep your neck in line with your spine, it may help to place a folded towel between your arm and head.) Bend your knees so your thighs form a 45-degree angle with your hips. Holding a light (2- to 5-pound) weight in your left hand, bend your left arm so your hand is by your ear and your elbow is pointing toward the ceiling. Exhale as you straighten the arm, lifting the weight toward the ceiling. Inhale as you lower the weight to the starting position. Repeat 8 to 12 times. Turn onto your left side and repeat with your right arm. If you feel up to it, work your way up to three sets.

Things to bear in mind: Keep your abs contracted throughout and your hips stacked. If you feel yourself rolling, place a pillow under your tummy and behind you for support. As you lift, keep your wrist in a neutral position.

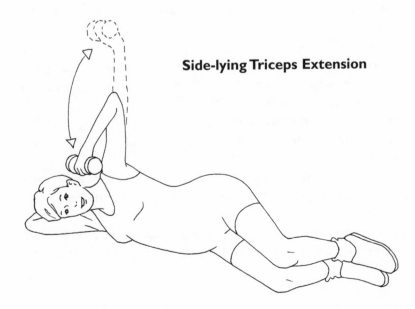

Side-lying Triceps Extension

ADVANCED KEGEL

Muscles it targets: Pubococcygeus, or PC muscle (see page 16).

Why do it: A strong pelvic floor is also a supple pelvic floor, which means it will stretch easier once it comes time to push your baby out.

How to do it correctly: Lie down on your left side or sit on the floor with your back against a wall, your legs slightly spread. Imagine that your pelvic floor is an elevator. To make it rise, you need to contract your pubococcygeus muscle bit by bit. To the count of five, contract your pelvic floor gradually with each subsequent number, until it's fully contracted by the time you reach number 5. Then gradually relax the muscle, allowing it to "descend," as if it were an elevator, back to the starting position. When you reach the starting position, focus on slackening and relaxing the muscle even further.

Things to bear in mind: Keep breathing naturally throughout the move. Don't hold your breath.

How to Cope with Navel Pain

It's astounding to realize how many minor complaints are associated with something so miraculous as pregnancy. You might expect your back to ache or your abdomen to get uncomfortable, but your *belly button*? Is nothing sacred?

Apparently not. Until now, you've probably been somewhat amused to mark your pregnancy's progress by the changes in your navel. Especially if you started with an "inny," it can be amazing to see it stretched flat by the growth of your belly. As your uterus continues to expand, however, prepare yourself: Your belly button may actually start to protrude outward, and this pregnancy-related "outy" can be surprisingly uncomfortable, causing everything from weird twinges to irritating skin sensitivity. For many women, even the friction from a favorite cotton T-shirt feels unpleasant by the end of this trimester.

Here's what to do to soothe an aching navel:

• Ice it. Wrap several ice cubes in a washcloth and hold it on the sore spot for a minute or two.

• Cover it up, especially when you exercise. A regular old bandage can provide a buffer between your popped-out belly button and a sweaty T-shirt or pregnancy tights that might rub it the wrong way.

• Work your abs. Strong abdominal muscles give your navel more support, which can help prevent some of the crampy kind of pulling sensations in the area.

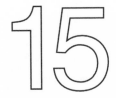

15 Enhancing Flexibility

Backaches. Insomnia. Swelling. Heartburn. By now the litany of pregnancy ailments is familiar. Although you've probably discovered that cardiovascular and strengthening exercises can go a long way toward providing relief, they're only part of the prescription. You have to stretch, too. If you haven't been doing so up to now, this is a perfect time to start focusing on flexibility, since stretches are the easiest form of exercise. If you have been diligent about setting aside some time to stretch, give yourself a big pat on the back. Now we want you to redouble your efforts to make flexibility work a part of your daily routine. Sneak a stretch or two in anytime, anyplace you get the chance.

We recommend you continue doing the moves from the routine we outlined in chapter 7. In addition, we've added some special third-trimester stretches that will help you prepare for labor and avoid some of the possible nastier late-pregnancy occurrences like sciatica, low back pain, and calf cramps. You don't have to do every single stretch every day if you don't feel up to it. But try to do at least five moves targeting various body parts, particularly anything that feels painful, tight, achy, or swollen.

As your due date draws near, you may find your regular exercise routine falling by the wayside. It's okay to slack off in the sweating department if you're simply feeling too big and tired to lumber through a full cardiovascular or strength routine. But don't give up on stretching. In fact, it's a great time to make flexibility the focus of your training regimen. It's a gentle, manageable way to get your muscles moving, and it can keep your body supple and tension-free as you await D-day.

How to Cope with Sciatica

It may have occurred to you that pregnancy is a pain in the butt. If you have sciatica, that sentiment is all too accurate.

Sciatica is actually pain in the sciatic nerve, your body's largest, running from your pelvis all the way down the backs of your legs to your feet. The swelling, postural changes, and pressure from your enlarging uterus can irritate this nerve, causing the buttock and leg pain characteristic of sciatica. Although symptoms can be exacerbated by running, lifting, and deep bending, you may have problems if you do none of those things; likewise, you may avoid the problem entirely even if you're a regular runner.

One way to prevent sciatica is to strengthen your abdominal muscles, which work in opposition to those that run along the back of the spine by the sciatic nerve. Resting on a firm mattress can alleviate the symptoms, as can the following stretch, which you can do with the help of a partner:

Lie on the floor on the side that doesn't hurt. Raise the knee of the upper leg to waist level, so your femur is perpendicular to your body. Then, allow the knee to drop to the floor in front of your body. Have your partner hold the knee down with one hand while he gently lifts the ankle of the same leg with the other hand. He should lift only an inch or two or as far as is comfortable. Hold the stretch for 20 seconds. Repeat three times.

SUPPORTED HIP SWAY

Muscles it targets: Pelvic, hip, and lower back muscles.

Why do it: To relieve tension in the lower back and relax the pelvis. This motion can provide some relief during labor as well.

How to do it correctly: Stand with your feet hip-distance apart and your knees relaxed. Holding onto a bed frame, doorjamb, or other stationary object for support, bend forward slightly at the waist and swing your hips slowly from side to side.

When to do it: Anytime you feel back or pelvic discomfort, after a long period of sitting or standing, during labor.

FULL BACK STRETCH

Muscles it targets: Delts, rhomboids, lats, and erector spinae.

Why do it: To lengthen your spine and back muscles and ease upper and lower back tension.

How to do it correctly: Stand with your feet hip-distance apart and your knees relaxed. Holding onto a bed frame, doorjamb, or other stationary object for support, bend your knees and round your back, tucking your chin toward your chest and your pelvis under. Feel the stretch along the length of your spine. Hold the stretch.

When to do it: After a workout, after a day of sitting or standing, anytime you feel lower back discomfort.

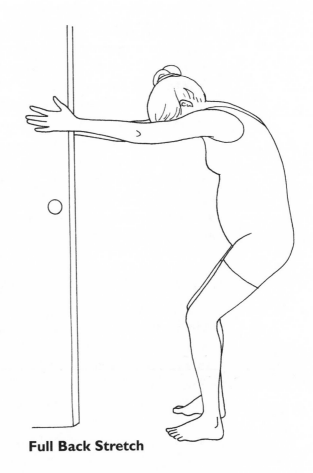

Full Back Stretch

TAILOR STRETCH

Muscles it targets: Inner thigh, hips, and pelvic floor.

Why do it: To encourage the widening of your pelvis, improve flexibility in your hip joints, and relax the pelvic floor muscles in preparation for labor.

How to do it correctly: Sitting on your butt bones, bend both knees and bring the soles of your feet together in front of you. Place a pillow underneath each knee to support your legs. Allow your feet to rest a comfortable distance from your body. Sit up tall, feeling a gentle stretch in your spine as well as your legs. Hold.

When to do it: After working out, before bed at night.

CHILD'S KNEEL

Muscles it targets: Pelvic, quadriceps, and back muscles.

Why do it: To open your pelvis and chest and lengthen your spine.

How to do it correctly: Place a folded blanket or towel and a couple of pillows on the floor. Kneel on the blanket with the pillows between your legs, and allow your weight to drop onto the pillows so you feel grounded at the base of your spine. (Your toes should be turned inward toward the pillows.) Slowly raise your arms overhead, keeping your shoulders relaxed, your elbows soft, and your wrists loose. Hold for a count of ten. Repeat three times.

When to do it: After a workout, before bed at night, when you're watching TV.

CHILD'S POSE

Muscles it targets: Back and inner thigh muscles.

Why do it: To release tension in your pelvis and back and lengthen your spine.

How to do it correctly: Place a folded blanket or towel and a couple of pillows on the floor. Kneel on the blanket with the pillows between your legs, and allow your weight to drop onto the pillows so you feel grounded at the base of your spine. (Your toes should be turned inward toward the pillows.) Raise your arms overhead, then slowly lower your torso forward to the ground so your arms are extended and your palms are flat on the floor in front of you. As you inhale, feel your spine lengthen. As you exhale, feel your chest release toward the floor. Hold for a count of ten.

When to do it: After a workout, before bed at night, when you're watching TV.

Child's Pose

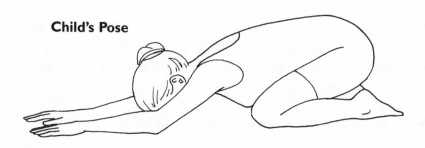

CALF, FOOT, AND ANKLE STRETCH

Muscles it targets: Calves, the arch of your foot, and the tendons and ligaments surrounding your ankle.

Why do it: To prevent calf cramps, to enhance range of motion in your ankles, and to improve circulation in your legs.

How to do it correctly: Sitting on the floor with your back against a wall for support, stretch your legs out in front of you. Wiggle your toes. Then push out through your heels, flexing your toes back toward you as you do so. Hold the stretch. Then spread your legs about 2 feet apart and circle your feet around to the outside 10 times, then to the inside 10 times.

When to do it: When you wake up in the morning, after a workout, before bed at night.

How to Cope with Leg Cramps

You've finally gotten to sleep after several hours of trying to find a comfortable position, then—wham!—you're awakened by an excruciating calf cramp. These painful spasms, which also may occur during exercise or (heaven help us) sex, are more common in pregnant women than in the population at large, possibly because pregnant women are more likely to get too little calcium or magnesium.

A random leg cramp is nothing to worry about, but if you're getting a lot of them, be sure your diet contains adequate calcium (see chapter 3 for recommendations) or talk to your doctor about taking calcium or magnesium supplements. A Swedish study found that oral magnesium may reduce the severity of leg cramps, but you should never take it without the express permission of your doctor. You might also try taking a warm bath or stretching your calves (see above) before you go to bed at night, both of which relax the muscles.

What to do when a calf cramp strikes:
• Stretch the leg straight out and gently flex your toes back toward your nose, which should relax the muscles that have tensed up.
• Ask your partner to gently push on the ball of the foot with the palm of his hand to lightly stretch your calf.
• Once the worst of the pain has passed, have your partner massage the calf muscles lightly in a circular motion, or apply a heating pad to the area to soothe the muscles.

recovering your body

Your Changing Body

Cardiovascular Fitness

Getting Stronger

Enhancing Flexibility

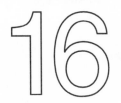

Your Changing Body

If you're like most anxious mothers-to-be, you've skipped ahead and are reading this while you're still pregnant. That's okay. It's not a bad idea to know what you're in for. Besides, you probably have more time on your hands prebaby than postbaby. If you actually waited, though, and you're snatching a little alone time while your new cherub is napping— first of all, congratulations! Second, sit back, try to relax, and think about some of the following issues that arise in the after-birth period.

For instance, you may be starting to realize just how much you *don't* know about how to care for yourself in the days and weeks after giving birth. In a study published in the journal *Birth,* researchers surveyed more than 540 first-time mothers and 621 mothers who already had children, at 7 weeks postpartum. They found that, while many women felt they could use more information on how to care for their baby, they were surprisingly uncertain about self-care.

The number one concern that first-time mothers wanted to have addressed was self-care in the area of exercise, diet, and nutrition. Nearly half felt they needed more information on those topics, while 44 percent wanted to learn more about fatigue, and 42 percent were confused about when they could resume normal activities. Of the experienced mothers, 40 percent said they needed more exercise information, 34 percent wanted to know more about fatigue, and nearly 28 percent wanted to know when to resume normal activities.

In this chapter we've tried to fill that information gap by providing the basics and answering your most pressing questions about how to nurture yourself in this exciting, exhausting, unbelievable new era of parenthood.

The truth is, recuperating from labor and delivery is a little bit like trying to move a mountain one cupful of dirt at a time . . . in a high wind . . . blindfolded. We could go on, but you get the point. You're trying to recover from a physical ordeal that's left you with all the energy of a garden snail, *and* you have a number of factors working against you— namely, little or no sleep, copious bleeding from a certain sensitive orifice, and an unusually demanding new job that gives you precious little time to brush your teeth, much less nurse yourself back to health. All of which may be compounded by a vague but inescapable anxiety stemming from the fact that you are now somebody's mother.

No matter what amazing physical feats you've accomplished in your past—summitting mountains, running rapids, completing marathons—the early weeks after having a baby will surely rank right up there with the most arduous. If you're nursing, tack on an additional degree of difficulty. If you have round-the-clock help (lucky you!), your life may be somewhat easier, but we'd wager you're still not sitting around eating bonbons and watching daytime talk shows. With the need for hourly diaper changes, dozens of feedings, daily baths, and near-constant cuddling and comforting, a baby could easily keep a whole army of attentive caregivers hustling.

How is exercise supposed to fit into this overcrowded schedule? Perhaps more importantly, do we actually expect you to resume physical activity *now*? Well, yes and no. We're not recommending that you spring off the delivery bed and do a lap around the hospital. In fact, depending on how you feel, we think it's a good idea for you to take anywhere from a few days to a whole week before even attempting to walk around the block. That said, most experts now agree you don't have to wait until your six-week checkup to start a rudimentary exercise program. (Check out chapters 17, 18, and 19 for specifics on cardiovascular, strength, and flexibility exercises.)

Some of you genuine fitness zealots may think that's the best news you've heard all year. But others (maybe the majority) of you may be thinking, "Great, one more thing for the to-do list." It's true that exercise does take a little time, and, with everything that's going on in your life right now, it certainly would be easier to just skip it. But the benefits that exercise provides make a pretty compelling case for getting started as soon as you feel able.

Getting physical will not only help you lose weight and tone up, but may also speed your healing. Starting your Kegel exercises in the days

How to Cope with a Cesarean

If recovering from a regular labor and delivery is difficult, bouncing back after a C-section is even more so. Like it or not, you've had major abdominal surgery, and you're going to need to give yourself extra time to recuperate, not just in the hospital but at home as well. Here's how to make your recovery as painless as possible:

• Enlist the help of everyone who offers. You should be resting as much as you can, especially during the first several weeks, so whenever possible let other people cook, tidy the house, change the baby's diaper, even make phone calls.

• Ease your pain. If your doctor prescribes medicine or suggests an over-the-counter analgesic, take it as directed. You'll feel better—maybe even recover more quickly—if you're in less pain.

• Contract your abs. Although actual crunches may be a month or two away for you, you can start gentle, static abdominal contractions while lying on your back in the hospital. Not only will it begin toning the area, it may promote healing around your incisions by increasing blood flow to the area.

• Move into exercise slowly. Although conventional wisdom holds that you can start easy stretching exercises and slow walking at about two weeks and begin a more strenuous program at five weeks, check with your doctor to be sure. Then watch for signs that you're doing too much. If you feel dizzy, faint, or nauseated, or if the incision from your C-section pulls or hurts with exertion, stop exercising.

• Rock away your gas. To banish the painful trapped gas that can accumulate in your gut in the days and weeks following a C-section, rock in a rocking chair for half an hour two or three times a day. In order to reap the benefits of this technique, you need to push off the ground fairly vigorously.

immediately following your baby's birth, for instance, encourages healing of an episiotomy incision or tear by increasing blood flow to the area. Getting your abs back in shape can help protect your back during the endless hours of lifting and carrying that lie in your future. And carving out even a few minutes a day for exercise can give you an emotional lift during this trying period. (See "Your Postpregnancy Brain," page 163, for more details on your state of mind.)

Of course, there are some physical considerations you're going to need to factor into your exercise plan. We'll get to those in a minute. But before we take stock of your physical inventory, we'd like to give you some perspective on how long this whole getting-your-body-back project is likely to take. The short answer: longer than you think.

The six-week recovery myth is just that—a big, fat fiction that has done easily as much damage to women's self-esteem as airbrushed photographs of models and the invention of Lycra. If you're still laboring under the misconception that you're going to be back to normal in a mere forty-two days, it's time for a reality check. Although the superficial wounds of your body may be well on their way to healing by then, the deeper changes caused by pregnancy can linger for months after giving birth, as can those pregnancy pounds, and pesky problems—things like hair loss and frequent respiratory illnesses—may actually get *worse* after the first month or so.

One study that looked at ninety-six mothers of healthy, full-term infants six months after delivery found that 25 percent of them still did not feel physically recovered from childbirth. Their list of problems included fatigue, difficulty losing weight, and emotional lability (changeability).

Furthermore, researchers at the University of Minnesota followed 436 first-time mothers for a full year after they gave birth to assess the reality of postpartum recovery. They found that problems like fatigue, hemorrhoids, constipation, heavy sweating, acne, hand numbness or tingling, dizziness, and hot flashes were actually worse at one month than they had been immediately after delivery; vaginal discomfort persisted for nine months in some women and even a year after delivery for others; 20 percent of the women were having sexual problems, such as discomfort during intercourse, decreased desire, and difficulty reaching orgasm. Moreover, the percentage of women with at least one respiratory symptom rose from 25 percent at one month to 42 percent at three months postpartum and remained greater than 40 percent for the rest of the year.

Given that, we'd like you to substitute that nearly-impossible-to-meet six-week deadline with a more liberal give-it-a-year kind of attitude. Try to be patient with yourself. Keep the following physical alterations in mind as you start to become more active and let your body recover gradually. That way, you'll spend less time and energy obsessing about things that are largely out of your control and more time enjoying your motherhood. Before you know it, you'll be feeling and looking more like your old self.

Breast tenderness and breast-feeding Although breast tenderness is much more pronounced in women who are nursing, even non-nursing mothers can have up to a month or more of discomfort as their bodies adjust to the postpregnancy period. Wearing a tight, supportive bra, especially when you exercise, can help relieve any discomfort, as can ice packs and over-the-counter pain relievers like acetaminophen.

In a University of Minnesota study, nipple irritation and breast discomfort were common three months after delivery in the breast-feeding mothers but tapered off significantly by six months. In other words, if you'd envisioned yourself as this saintly, Madonna-esque mother serenely nursing her newborn, you might be in for a rude awakening in the first few weeks. Breast-feeding hurts, especially at first. No small wonder, since your little one uses your breasts as everything from food supply to a source of comfort. Although time is the best healer, there are some things you can do until your body gets used to being a "breastaurant":

• Make sure you have the baby positioned correctly and that he or she is latching on the right way. There are lots of breast-feeding books on the market that describe in detail how to breast-feed. If you're still not sure, ask your doctor for advice or call a lactation specialist.

• After nursing, express a little breast milk onto a clean fingertip and rub it around. Interestingly, this natural cure is still thought to be the best.

• Allow your breasts to air-dry after each nursing.

• Remove your athletic bra immediately after exercising to prevent chafing. If you're wearing nursing pads, moisten them with a little water before you remove them to prevent them from sticking to your nipples.

• Don't use soap on your breasts; it can be drying.

• Apply ice to your nipples between feedings and warm compresses right before feedings.

• Apply hypoallergenic lanolin to your nipples after feedings.

If you are breast-feeding, you should also expect to once again invest in some new athletic bras. If you didn't need them before, you almost certainly will now as your breasts swell with milk, which will happen two to four days after you give birth. You may be one or even two cup sizes larger than you were during pregnancy, and that extra voluptuousness can make exercising tricky thanks to the flop factor. One solution: Wear two exercise bras, one on top of the other, for extra support. Make sure they're the compression style, which works better for this technique than the lift-and-separate variety.

In addition, you'll need to plan your workouts around your nursing schedule, since recent studies have shown exercise can affect the content of your breast milk. Some researchers have found a small percentage of babies don't like the taste of postexercise breast milk, which contains more lactic acid than regular breast milk. Another study found concentrations of the immune-system booster IgA decreased for up to thirty minutes in the breast milk of women who exercised strenuously. IgA levels in breast milk returned to normal one hour after exercising. To make sure your baby is receiving the best-tasting, healthiest milk, try to nurse her or express some breast milk before you exercise, then wait up to an hour after exercising before nursing again.

You'll also need to be especially conscientious about getting enough fluids. Breast-feeding itself is a big fluid drain; add exercise to the picture, and you could easily be in for a case of dehydration. To avoid it, drink as much water as you can (see our tips in chapter 3). Have a glass of water every time you nurse the baby, and keep one handy while you're working out. To make sure you're staying well hydrated, monitor your urine. If it looks dark yellow or has a strong odor, you need to consume more fluids.

Joint laxity The effects of the hormone relaxin, which made your joints and ligaments all loosey-goosey during pregnancy, may linger for up to four months after you've had the baby—meaning you should still take care not to turn your ankle when you're walking, or not to overstretch. As a result, it's probably best to avoid activities that require lots of quick, explosive moves for the first few months after delivery. What does that mean if you're an avid tennis player? No one is saying you can't participate in sports you love. You just need to take it slowly and move with more awareness. Try to avoid big lunges and abrupt movements. In short, just be mindful of the fact that your body is somewhat less stable than it was in your prepregnancy days.

Vaginal pain Even if you didn't have an episiotomy, you're likely to be pretty sore in the days following delivery. If you did have an episiotomy or perineal tear, don't be surprised if that is the most agonizing aspect of your postpartum experience. Everything from getting out of bed to going to the bathroom can be excruciating in those first few days. To ease the pain, apply ice packs, take a warm sitz bath several times a day, then dry the area with a blow-dryer, and take acetaminophen.

The pain should start to abate within a week or so, but some women may still be quite uncomfortable two or even three weeks after delivery, and mild discomfort can last nine months or more. Let your comfort level dictate how quickly you return to aerobic activities like walking. Getting out in short spurts, rather than going for extended forays, is one way to fulfill your aerobic exercise needs without irritating your sensitive parts.

Bleeding You might expect your nether regions to be uncomfortable after delivering a baby, but, unless you have some really honest friends, you may be shocked at the amount of postdelivery "discharge"—the euphemism doctors use for the Niagara Falls–like blood flow you'll experience for the first week or so. Most often, the industrial-strength flow diminishes to a more normal menstrual-like quantity after four or five days and it changes in color from bright red to pink or brownish. But you may continue to bleed at least intermittently for up to eight weeks.

To cope with this astonishing outpouring, use extralarge sanitary pads, not tampons. They may be uncomfortable when you exercise, but they're safest. As you ease back into working out, keep tabs on the rate of your flow. If your bleeding increases or looks more red after exercise, it's a signal you're doing too much. Take it easy for a day or two to give your body time to adjust, then start again slowly. If you start bleeding even more heavily anytime after the first few days, to the point where you're soaking more than one sanitary pad an hour, call your doctor immediately.

Weakened abdominals When there was a baby inside pulling your muscles taut, it may have been hard to tell how much strength you'd actually lost. Now that the baby is on the outside, however, you've got ample opportunity to survey the damage. Let's face it: It's not pretty. Any activity requiring abdominal strength—getting out of bed or lifting the baby—is going to feel difficult. Which means your back is more vulnerable to injury since it's lacking one of its main support systems. Take care when lifting, and attempt to bear the brunt of the weight with your legs until you can get your abdominal muscles back in working order.

Although much of your body will return to normal without your conscious help, your abs are a notable exception. Unless you make some effort, they will remain weak and stretched out. The good news is you can start to rehab your abs immediately. Anytime you feel up to it within the first five days of giving birth (the sooner the better), we suggest you start consciously sucking in your abdominal muscles, like you would if you'd just walked out in your bikini onto the deck of a crowded swimming pool.

You can start doing real crunches once your diastasis is largely gone. To check, lie on your back with your knees bent and your feet flat on the floor about a foot apart. Place the fingers of your right hand on your belly just above your belly button so your fingers form a vertical line along your midsection. Slowly raise your head and shoulders. As you do so, you should feel a band of muscles on either side of your fingers. Those are your recti muscles. Almost all postpartum women will have a gap between the recti. (It won't protrude now, since your uterus isn't full.) If your gap is large—more than two finger widths—you'll need to do modified crunches before you do regular ones. Here's how:

Lie on your back with your knees bent and your feet flat on the floor about a foot apart. Wrap your arms around your belly so your hands are resting on opposite sides of your waist. Exhale as you lift your head (not your shoulders) off the floor, pulling your recti muscles together with your hands as you do so. Release and repeat. Work your way up to 40 a day.

How to Cope with Urinary Incontinence

You expected the baby to pee its pants on a regular basis, but you may be alarmed when you realize that every time you cough, sneeze, exercise, or perform any high-impact activity you may have your own problems to contend with.

Though most of us associate urinary incontinence with the blue-hair-and-bingo set, the problem strikes at least one in ten women under the age of sixty-five and is quite common among mothers, especially those who had large babies or who pushed for more than three hours during delivery. The reason: Labor and delivery not only strain your pubococcygeus and other pelvic floor muscles directly but also stretch the nerves inside those muscles, which weakens the muscles even further. Moreover, when you bear down during the final stages of labor, you stretch the connective tissues that support the bladder and urethra, causing those organs to sag and exert even more pressure on the pelvic floor muscles.

For some women, the problem resolves itself within a few months, as the pelvic floor muscles naturally regain their strength. Others may need to put in some extra effort to get their bodies under control. Here are things that can help:
• Do your Kegel exercises. Those contract and release moves we've had you doing since day one of pregnancy are the best first line of intervention for postpartum stress incontinence. Experts estimate that, when done regularly and properly, Kegels can significantly reduce the problem in at least half of the women who have it. You should notice a difference in about six weeks, but optimal effect takes about three months. If you don't get results from Kegels, it could be that you're doing them wrong. Check with your doctor to be sure you're doing them correctly. If you're not, a session or two of biofeedback can help you learn to Kegel properly.
• Add some weight to your Kegel workout. Vaginal cones are cone-shaped weights that fit into the vagina. When you Kegel with a weight in, you build muscle strength more quickly.
• To minimize the problem, cut your consumption of coffee, tea, and caffeinated soda, all of which are diuretics that make you urinate more than you normally would.
• If you're overweight, shed some pounds. Excess weight means excess pressure on the bladder.
• Try a technique called "bladder retraining." For one week, put yourself on a strict peeing schedule, visiting the bathroom at least once an hour. Then, increase the time between potty stops by 15 to 20 minutes to force your pelvic floor muscles into action. By learning to hold back the flow, the theory goes, you're retraining your muscles to do their job.
• If all else fails, surgery can often correct the problem.

Keep checking your diastasis periodically. Once the gap between the recti muscles is less than two finger widths, you can resume regular crunches.

Sweating and urinating During pregnancy you accumulated an unbelievable amount of fluid in your system, and now it's going to come pouring out of every orifice, leaving you drenched at night and running to the bathroom all day. There's not a lot to do about this annoyance but ride it out. After a few weeks, your fluid levels should stabilize. Sweating during exercise may help clear some of this excess fluid from your body sooner. Just be sure to keep downing the water. All that peeing doesn't mean you should cut back on consumption.

Extra weight In the first few hours after you have the baby, you're going to feel skinny because you won't have that hard watermelon belly hanging off your torso. Besides, you probably lost about 12 pounds in the course of a few hours—undoubtedly the speediest weight-loss program around. But here's the biggest downer after pregnancy: Even a week or two (or more) after delivery, someone may ask you when you're expecting. You still look *that* pregnant. The lump under your shirt may be as squishy as Play-Doh, but it's still a lump, and it can be quite a sizable one.

There are several reasons for this postpartum affront to your figure. First, your uterus is still enlarged. It probably won't shrink and drop back into its rightful place in your pelvis until about six weeks after delivery. Meanwhile, for the first week or so you're also bloated with extra pregnancy fluids, and for at least a month or two, you won't have the abdominal strength to suck in your gut.

If you can't stand the sight of your maternity clothes but can't wriggle your way into your prepregnancy stuff, snatch big shirts from your partner's closet and invest in a pair or two of comfortable leggings. For workouts, wear what fits. Big T-shirts can hide anything that skimpy Lycra shorts would dare to expose.

You'll definitely notice those extra pounds as you start to resume normal activities, and they'll feel especially onerous when you do weight-bearing exercise. Take care to work within your limitations, and don't expect your postpartum body to perform like your prepregnancy one.

How long will it take you to lose those extra pounds? That depends on a number of factors, like how much weight you gained during pregnancy, how active you are, what your diet is like, and if you are breast-feeding or not. For the first six weeks, it's not a good idea for anyone to restrict calories, because your body is trying to heal. You need calories to fuel your recovery. If you're breast-feeding, it's especially critical that you eat well, because your milk production is being established—a process that requires lots of energy.

Even without dieting, your body will shed weight naturally (assuming you don't *overeat*) over the course of the next several months. Breast-feeding women tend to lose weight at an average rate of about 1.5 pounds per month during the first four to six months, but some women, breast-feeding or not, may lose up to 4 pounds a month for the first several months. In general, experts say you shouldn't strive to lose weight any more quickly than that, because rapid weight loss can sap your energy and decrease your milk supply if you're breast-feeding. Also, if you're breast-feeding, expect to hang onto 3 to 5 extra pounds for months. Although some women drop to their prepregnancy weight while nursing, many find those last few pounds resist their best efforts until they wean their babies.

Although exercise will help you in your quest to return to your prepregnancy shape, it won't offset overconsumption. The winning (or should we say losing?) combination: regular exercise paired with a healthful, moderate diet.

Nutrition After Pregnancy

After adding pounds for nine months, you're probably anxious to start shedding them. As a result, you may be tempted to toss all those healthy pregnancy eating habits out the window in favor of some gimmicky weight-loss plan promising speedy results. Now hear this: Starvation diets aren't for new mothers. Moms need energy, and lots of it, so moms need calories, especially if they're breast-feeding. As some wise person once said, you can't spell the word *healthy* without the letters *E, A, T.* Depending on your build and activity level, you should consume anywhere from 1,800 to 2,500 calories per day if you're breast-feeding, and 1,500 to 2,000 calories per day if you're formula-feeding.

That doesn't mean you should overeat. In a Swedish study of 1,423 postpartum women, 57 percent of women weighed 2 to 11 pounds more than their prepregnancy weight one year after they'd had a baby. The researchers attributed their weight gain to two primary factors: too little physical activity and too many snacks. Women who retained weight tended to skip lunch and eat three or more snacks a day.

A good rule of thumb is to let your rate of weight loss dictate how much you eat. If you're losing more than a pound a week you need to eat more. If your scale hasn't budged since delivery, it's safe—even advisable—for you to cut back your calories slightly.

Counting calories is only half the battle, however. What you eat is equally important if you want to recover quickly and have enough energy to enjoy your baby. Fortunately, you've had nine months of nutrition training, so this healthy eating thing is old hat by now. In general, a healthy postpartum diet looks a lot like a pregnancy diet, with a few special considerations. For the first couple of weeks, you'll need to pay extra attention to your iron and fluid consumption, since you'll be bleeding fairly heavily. In addition, you'll want a full complement of the nutrients that help your body combat stress, the most noteworthy being folic acid and vitamin B_6 as well as vitamin C, which promotes healing and aids in iron absorption.

If you're breast-feeding, you need an extra serving or two of calcium every day since studies have shown that calcium can be leached from your bones if you don't consume enough to fuel milk production. To make sure you're meeting your needs, expand your calcium-rich repertoire to include foods like sardines, dark green vegetables, and tofu. You should also try to get at least three servings of protein a day, and drink plenty of fluids, even if you don't feel thirsty.

Your Postpregnancy Brain

Even if you're thrilled to bits to be a mommy, your diet is so exemplary you could be a poster child for the American Dietetic Association, and your body is healing nicely, there are going to be days (maybe lots of them) when you feel something less than functional—when the idea of facing another poopy diaper seems almost unbearable; when you marvel at the fact that you were once able to hold an intelligent conversation about global warming or stock prices or a current movie; when you wonder if you'll ever have anything resembling a social life (or sex life) again.

Fear not. You're not a freak or an unfit parent. You're simply adjusting to the onslaught of physical and emotional changes a new baby brings. Not only are you contending with a mood-altering drop in estrogen and progesterone in the postbirth period, but you're also grappling with sleep deprivation, new responsibilities and stressors, and diminished physical capacities, at least in the short term.

It's probably some combination of these factors that accounts for the whopping 70 percent of women who experience postpartum blues, a weepy, irritable episode lasting three to five days, typically during the first week after delivery. Those factors are also the most likely culprits in postpartum depression, a disorder characterized by crying, irritability, apathy, anxiety, lack of appetite, inability to sleep, and highly impaired concentration and decision making. It strikes an estimated 10 to 15 percent of women in their first year after giving birth, typically beginning in the first three months. Doctors say if you have the symptoms of postpartum depression for at least two weeks, you should seek professional help.

Most transient moodiness doesn't require medical attention, but it does call for some added TLC. To boost your spirits, get a massage, have dinner with a friend (but leave the baby home with your husband), sleep any chance you get, and accept any and all offers of help. And deploy your secret mood-boosting weapon: exercise. A study published in the *Journal of Sports Medicine and Physical Fitness* found 60 minutes of low-impact aerobic activity decreased depression, anxiety, and general mood disturbances and increased physical vigor in women who had given birth in the previous year.

Fitness Q & A

1

I had my baby two months ago, and I'm still utterly exhausted. Is it healthy to exercise when you barely have the energy to comb your hair?

Yes, if you define the term "exercise" fairly loosely. Pushing yourself through a whole aerobics class or typical prepregnancy workout may be too much right now, but it can be beneficial—and energy-enhancing—to take easy walks or swims. One simple guideline should help ensure you don't do too much: End your workout when you're still feeling energized.

If you're worried there's something abnormal about your fatigue, get a medical checkup. A condition like iron-deficiency anemia could be contributing to your woes. But chances are you're not suffering from anything more serious than New Parent Syndrome, the unofficial scourge of all new mothers.

Every morning I resolve to exercise, and every night I go to bed without having squeezed it in. Just exactly when is a new mother supposed to find the time to work out?

Good question. Despite most women's fervent desire to return to their prepregnancy shapes, it wouldn't be surprising if more gym memberships lapse in the postpartum period than at any other time. Caring for an infant requires nearly every available second, and it's the rare woman who isn't stymied by the time conundrum. Following are a few suggestions to help you find the time:

• Break up your workout into small manageable chunks. Go for a walk before your husband leaves for work in the morning, sneak out for a short stroll when friends and relatives visit, do a few crunches during the baby's naptime. The latest research shows the piecemeal approach is every bit as effective as the all-at-once method.

• Get your baby into the act. Put your baby in a front pack or sling and do some lunges or pliés (we offer more exercise-with-baby suggestions in chapter 18), or go for a walk. The extra weight makes it a better workout, and the rhythmic motion will probably lull your little one to sleep. Jog strollers are a great way to get exercise, too. Just be sure your baby is shielded from the sun and adequately bundled. The faster you go, the more wind chill there will be on the baby.

• Put on some music and dance with your baby. You'll rediscover what good exercise simple *movement* can be.

• Set priorities. Your abdominals are undoubtedly your most lackluster muscles these days thanks to what they've been through recently, so give them attention before, say, your biceps, which are getting a fair amount of work already.

• Cut out time wasters. When you actually steal a few moments to do some strength training or stretching moves, don't dawdle between exercises. If you move from one to the next quickly, you can cram a good workout into a tight time slot.

• Once you're feeling up to it, increase the intensity of your cardio work. If you can't spend more time, this is the best way to get more for your (precious) minutes.

3 *My weight seems to be all over the map. One day I've lost a pound, the next day I've gained two. It's making me crazy! What's up?*

You've just discovered one of the most frustrating things about weight loss: It ain't linear. Things like fluid retention, a big meal, recent exercise, and dehydration can make the scale seem as unpredictable as your baby's sleeping schedule. Instead of falling prey to daily scale anxiety, weigh yourself once a week when you first wake up in the morning—pre-breakfast, preexercise. Don't wear any clothes and skip it the week before your period (if you're menstruating), when fluid retention can make it look like you've added pounds. Also, don't weigh yourself the morning after you've had too much alcohol or caffeine, both of which can be dehydrating and make your weight deceptively low. If you follow these tips, you'll almost surely see a slow but steady downward progression—and feel better about your body to boot.

4 *After my sister stopped nursing her daughter, her breasts actually became smaller than they were before she got pregnant. Does that happen to everyone, and, if so, is there anything you can do about it?*

No, it doesn't happen to everyone, but the double whammy of small *and* saggy strikes many post-breast-feeding women. Here's why: The breast tissue actually becomes less dense when you stop nursing, making breasts softer and droopier. Although there's not much you can do to firm up the connective tissue that once made your breasts perkier, you can improve the appearance of your bosom by building up your pecs, the underlying muscles supporting the area. Perhaps the single best pec exercise is the classic push-up, performed either on your knees or military style. This might also be a good time to invest in some new bras. There are lots of styles on the market that will give you the lift you're looking for.

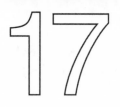

Cardiovascular Fitness

Even if you're carrying 20 extra pounds, getting active is going to feel so much easier now than it did when you were lugging a baby around in your belly. And if you exercised throughout your pregnancy, you may be thrilled to find you haven't lost much in the way of heart fitness. Still, that doesn't mean you should expect to be competing in a 10K at the one-month mark. Yes, there are women who make those kinds of miraculous recoveries, and if you find that inspiring, feel free to seek those stories out. We're not going to relate any here, though, and here's why: Most women are overly hard on themselves, and those "she-had-a-baby-one-day-and-was-out-running-the-next" anecdotes are likely to make you set unrealistically high standards for yourself, thereby setting yourself up for failure. Who needs that kind of pressure?

Instead, we're going to look at what most people are capable of doing, which, in the early days, isn't a heckuva lot. You're going to be sore, tired, and emotionally overwhelmed. In addition, time is going to feel like it's taken on a life of its own. Whole days are going to pass by and you won't know where they went. You may find the sun setting and realize you haven't made it out of your pajamas yet. Even control freaks are out of their league once they're in newborn land.

Given that, how should you approach exercise? With a good deal of flexibility and forgiveness. On page 168, we offer a safe, effective walking routine you can do outside or on a treadmill. Either way, it will get your fitness back on track by week 12 or so. Not into walking? There are any number of ways you can get back into the swing of things. (See "When You Can Do the Sports You Love," page 170, for some general guidelines.)

The golden rule: Some activity is better than none—unless, of course, you were up every hour on the hour all night, in which case we'd recommend you get some shut-eye at the earliest opportunity (no rule is set in stone). Life with baby is nothing if not unpredictable. So make exercise a goal, a priority, even. But don't give yourself twenty lashes if you miss a day (or a week). Let it be something you do for yourself, not because you have to but because you want to. If you can cultivate that mind-set, you'll find ways to fit it in, and you may even find the key to a lifelong commitment to fitness.

Gearing Up: The First Four Weeks

Depending on how you're faring, sometime within the first week to ten days we'd like you to go out for a walk. (If you had a C-section, check with your doctor before starting any exercise program.) It's the easiest, most convenient exercise around, and, if you own a good stroller or front carrier, it's one you can do with your baby. Aim for 5 minutes. If you feel okay, go for 10. Watch for the following signs of overexertion:
• An increase in bleeding or a change in its color from brownish to bright red
• Dizziness, faintness, or nausea
• Joint pain
• Exhaustion

If you weather that first outing well, try to do it again in a day or two, and then again a day or two after that. You should be walking at a leisurely 3 to 3.5 miles per hour—a pace at which you can easily carry on a conversation. Follow the walking tips we offered in chapter 5 to get the most out of each workout. If you're pushing a stroller, don't worry about the arm movements.

the program: Warm up by walking slowly for 5 minutes. Gradually add to your walking time in 5-minute increments, so you work your way up to 20 minutes, three to five days a week by the fourth week postpartum.

Making Progress: The Second Four Weeks

Once your bleeding has stopped, or slowed to occasional spotting, you can increase the intensity and duration of your regimen. One great way to do that is with interval training, an idea we introduced in chapter 9. When you're walking at an easy-to-moderate pace, lean forward slightly from the ankles, not from the waist. As your pace increases, lean forward from the hips and slightly from the ankles, and take shorter, quicker steps.

the program: Warm up by walking 5 minutes at an easy, 3-mile-per-hour pace. Then walk for 1 minute at a fast pace—4 to 4.5 miles per hour. Alternate 5-minute periods of moderate walking (3 to 3.5 miles per hour) with 1-minute periods of fast walking until you've walked about 30 minutes. Walk slowly for a minute or two to cool down. As you feel ready, gradually begin to increase the periods of fast walking and decrease the periods of moderate walking.

Feeling Fit: Eight Weeks and Beyond

You're well on your way to attaining a good, strong fitness level, and you're probably ready to ratchet things up a notch. The key to knowing when you're ready: You have increased the intensity of the regimen above and you still have energy to spare at the end of your workout. At this point, we recommend walking with your baby in a front carrier of some sort. (Try lots on to find the one that has the most comfortable fit.) We think this is a good idea for a couple of reasons. First, you're going to want to add to the duration of your workouts, and it's hard to find that much time without the baby. In addition, adding the 10 to 15 pounds to your torso increases the weight-bearing factor, which adds more stress to your bones—a key way to prevent osteoporosis. Why not reap as many health benefits as you can in the shortest amount of time?

the program: Warm up by walking 5 minutes at an easy, 3-mile-per-hour pace. Then, walk at a 4- to 4.5-mile-per-hour pace for 30 minutes. If you feel fatigued and need a break, intersperse 1- or 2-minute moderate-pace periods throughout your workout, but try to sustain as fast a pace as you can. Add 5 minutes to the duration of your workout until you can walk for a full hour at the fast pace. Try to do this workout at least three days a week, with one 30-minute walk, one 45-minute walk, and one 60-minute walk. As your fitness improves, up the challenge by adding hills to your route.

When You Can Do the Sports You Love

There are far fewer rules in the postpartum period than there were when you were pregnant, but that doesn't mean there aren't a few. With any activity, you should watch for signs you're doing too much, and stop before you're exhausted. You need to have something left over for your baby. The following suggestions apply to women who've had vaginal births. If you had a C-section, consult your doctor for advice on when you can resume your activity of choice.

ACTIVITY	WHEN TO RESUME
Aerobics	Can start low-impact as soon as you feel up to it after the baby is two weeks old, high-impact once you've stopped bleeding and had your six-week checkup.
Aerobics, step	Wait until your joints and balance are back to normal at about 4 to 6 months.
Bicycling	Wait until your episiotomy has healed and you can sit comfortably on the seat.
Cross-country skiing	Can do before 4 to 6 months if you take shorter-than-normal strides, which are easier on your joints.
Golf	Can return to easy swinging as soon as you feel up to it after the baby is two weeks old. Save 18 holes for after your six-week checkup.
In-line skating	Can do before 4 to 6 months if you take short strides. Don't use in-line skates with a jog stroller because you may get up too much speed.
Rowing	Can return to gentle activity as soon as you feel up to it after the baby is two weeks old.
Running	Wait until you've stopped bleeding and you can hold back your urine.
Snowshoeing	Wait until you've stopped bleeding and you can hold back your urine.
Soccer	Wait until your joints and balance are back to normal, at about 4 to 6 months.
Softball	Wait until you've stopped bleeding and can hold back your urine.
Stair-stepping machine	Can return to an easy pace as soon as you feel up to it after the baby is two weeks old.
Tennis	Wait until your joints and balance are back to normal at about 4 to 6 months.
Volleyball	Wait until you've stopped bleeding and can hold back your urine.
Weight lifting	Wait until you've stopped bleeding.
Yoga	Can do some moves as soon as you feel up to it after the baby is two weeks old. Avoid big lunges until your joints are back to normal, at about 4 to 6 months.
Swimming	Wait until you've stopped bleeding.

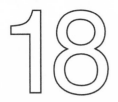

Getting Stronger

You may feel as weak as a kitten in the days following your delivery, but many of your muscles are as strong as they ever were—and some are maybe even stronger. Your legs, for instance, have supported lots of extra weight for the past few months, so they may be in top form, despite a little additional padding. Depending on how committed you were to exercising during your pregnancy, your arms, too, may be well muscled—a good thing, you'll find, since this is when you really need upper body strength.

Other muscles, however, most notably your abdominals and your pelvic floor, are destined to come out of pregnancy in pretty bad shape, and regaining the strength in those muscles is going to take some time and effort. Fortunately, you can begin to focus on toning those trouble spots from day one if you feel up to it.

On the following pages, you'll find a postpartum workout that starts with the easy stuff you can do right away, tells you when and how to progress, and puts you well on the road to a full-body recovery by 12 weeks. Since we know how hard it can be to sneak even a few solitary moments, most of the moves in our post-six-week workout can be done with or without baby. Welcome to the challenge of motherhood. We know you're up to the task.

BASIC KEGEL EXERCISES

Muscles it targets: Pubococcygeus, or PC muscle (see page 16).

Why do it: A strong pelvic floor helps prevent urinary stress incontinence and contributes to stronger orgasms.

How to do it correctly: In any position (lying on your back at first, then sitting up or standing), tighten your PC muscle and hold the contraction for 3 seconds. Do 8 to 12 reps. Work your way up to three sets.

Things to bear in mind: Keep breathing as you clench the muscle. To isolate the PC muscle, allow your abdominal and inner thigh muscles to relax.

TUMMY SUCK-IN

Muscles it targets: Abdominals.

Why do it: Your abs have been stretched out for nine months, and the only way to get them back into shape is exercise. This gentle toning work will help close up your diastasis and get your muscles ready for real crunches.

How to do it correctly: When you're lying on your back, imagine you're trying to pull your belly button in toward your spine. Do 8 to 12 reps. Work your way up to three sets.

Things to bear in mind: Don't hold your breath. Once you're up and around, be sure to hold in your abs every time you pick up the baby, walk, sit, or lie down.

SHOULDER BLADE SQUEEZE

Muscles it targets: Upper back muscles.

Why do it: To realign your spine and strengthen your back to help with the job of carrying the baby.

How to do it correctly: Sitting or standing, squeeze your shoulder blades toward each other. Do 8 to 12 reps. Work your way up to three sets.

Things to bear in mind: Keep your shoulders relaxed. Think "back and down" as you squeeze.

Continue doing the moves from the first two weeks and add:

OPPOSING LIFT

Muscles it targets: Back, abs, butt, and hamstrings.

Why do it: To regain your sense of balance and strengthen the back of your body.

How to do it correctly: Kneel on all fours with your knees directly under your hips and your arms directly under your shoulders. Simultaneously lift and extend your right leg behind you to hip height, and your right arm in front of you to shoulder height. Lower. Do 8 to 12 reps. Then switch sides.

Things to bear in mind: Lift and lower in a slow, controlled manner. No swinging! Keep your spine straight and your head in line with your spine.

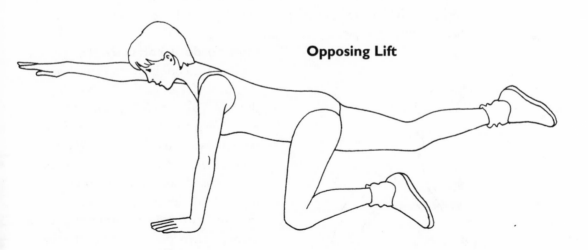

Opposing Lift

Weeks 4 to 6

Continue doing the previous moves. Check to see if you have a diastasis (see chapter 16, page 159, for a description of how to do it).

If your diastasis is smaller than two finger widths, add:
BASIC CRUNCH (see chapter 6, page 72)

If your diastasis is larger than two finger widths, add:
MODIFIED CRUNCH (see chapter 16, page 159)

Weeks 6 and Beyond

Continue Kegels and Tummy Suck-ins. Start the following workout when you feel up to it.

PUMPING BABY

Muscles it targets: Traps, lats, glutes, and hamstrings.
Why do it: To strengthen your upper back and legs, and to get in the habit of lifting properly.

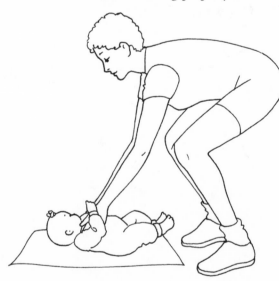

Pumping Baby

How to do it correctly: Lay your baby on the floor in front of you. Stand in front of her with your feet hip-distance apart. Bending your knees, reach down toward the baby. Bend from the hips with your back flat. Grab the baby under the armpits, with the palms of your hands supporting her neck and head. Slowly lift her, pulling her close to your body and using your legs for support. Then lower her to the floor by bending your knees and bending over at the hips, touch her rear to the floor, and lift her again. Do 8 to 12 reps.
Things to bear in mind: Breathe throughout the move. Keep your spine as straight as you can and pull your abs in firmly. Don't drop the baby.

TOE RAISE

Muscles it targets: Calves.

Why do it: To strengthen your calves for walking, running, etc.

How to do it correctly: With the baby in a front carrier, stand next to a wall, feet about hip-distance apart. Place your right hand on the wall for support. Then slowly raise yourself up onto your toes and lower. Do 8 to 12 reps. Work your way up to three sets.

Things to bear in mind: Add reps slowly. If you feel your calves tightening, stop and stretch.

CHAIR SQUAT

Muscles it targets: Glutes, quadriceps, and hamstrings.

Why do it: To firm up your backside and strengthen your quads for everyday activities.

How to do it correctly: With the baby in a front carrier, stand with your back to the seat of a chair, feet hip-distance apart. Bending your knees, slowly lower your butt toward the chair as if you were going to sit down. Keep your back straight. When your hamstrings skim the chair, return to the starting position. Do 8 to 12 reps. Work your way up to three sets.

Things to bear in mind: Keep your abs pulled in firmly and your weight in your heels as you squat.

TRICEPS DIP

Muscles it targets: Triceps.

Why do it: To build muscle in your arms and stave off the jiggle factor.

How to do it correctly: With the baby in a front carrier, sit on the edge of a firm chair that's backed up to a wall for support. (Be sure to wear nonskid footwear.) Place your feet flat on the floor about 2 feet in front of the chair, so your knees form a 90-degree angle and your thighs are parallel to the floor. With your palms on the front edge of the chair for support, drop your weight off the edge of the seat. Slowly bend your elbows to lower your butt toward the floor. Dip about 6 inches. Straighten

Triceps Dip

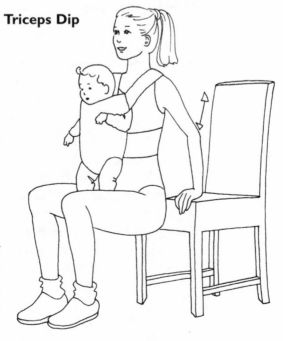

your arms to lift yourself back up so your butt is parallel to the seat. Do 8 to 12 reps. Work your way up to three sets.

Things to bear in mind: Don't hold your breath. Keep your body straight and close to the edge of the chair.

SEATED LAT ROW

Muscles it targets: Lats and rear delts.

Why do it: To get your upper back in shape for lifting.

How to do it correctly: With the baby on the floor in front of you in a bouncy seat or lying on a blanket, sit on the edge of a firm chair with your feet flat on the floor about 2 feet in front of the chair, so your knees form a 90-degree angle and your thighs are parallel to the floor. Holding a light weight in each hand, bend forward so your chest is nearly resting against your thighs and your arms are dangling on either side of your legs, palms facing your body. Pulling your shoulder blades together, bend your elbows until the weights are hip height. Return to the starting position. Do 8 to 12 reps. Work your way up to three sets.

Things to bear in mind: Keep your elbows close to your body as you lift. Concentrate on the contraction in your upper back.

SHOULDER PRESS

Muscles it targets: Pecs and delts.

Why do it: To build up your chest muscles and improve the appearance of your breast area.

How to do it correctly: With the baby on the floor in front of you in a bouncy seat or lying on a blanket, sit on the edge of a firm chair with your feet flat on the floor about 2 feet in front of the chair, so your knees form a 90-degree angle and your thighs are parallel to the floor. Holding a light weight in each hand, lift your arms out to the sides and bend your elbows 90 degrees, so your hands are up in the air, your palms facing forward. This is your starting position. Pull your arms together so the forearms meet in front. Return to the starting position. Do 8 to 12 reps. Work your way up to three sets.

Things to bear in mind: Feel the contraction in your chest. Continue breathing throughout the movement.

BUTT TUCK

Muscles it targets: Glutes.

Why do it: To keep your fanny toned.

How to do it correctly: Start on all fours with your thighs perpendicular to the floor, your back flat, and the baby lying beneath you on a blanket. Slowly tuck your tailbone under, squeezing your buttocks together as you tilt your pelvis. Hold for 3 seconds. Return to the starting position. Exhale as you tuck; inhale as you release. Do 8 to 12 reps. Work your way up to three sets.

Things to bear in mind: Don't let your lower back arch when you're in the starting position.

PUSH-UP

Muscles it targets: Pecs, front part of your delts, and triceps.

Why do it: To improve the appearance of your chest area and strengthen your upper body.

How to do it correctly: Start on all fours with your thighs perpendicular to the floor, your back flat, and the baby lying beneath you on a blanket. Slowly walk your hands forward so your knees are behind your hips and your weight is resting on your hands. Keeping your spine straight, inhale and bend your elbows and lower yourself down to rub noses with your baby. Exhale and return to the starting position. Do 8 to 12 reps. Work your way up to three sets.

Things to bear in mind: Keep your head in line with your spine.

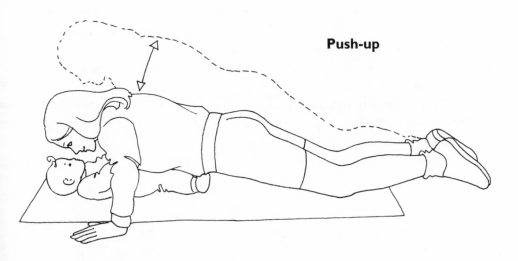

Push-up

SIDE-LYING OUTER THIGH LIFT

Muscles it targets: Outer hip and thigh muscles (aka abductors).

Why do it: To rehab your pelvic region.

How to do it correctly: Lie on your right side with your head resting comfortably on your right arm. (To keep your neck in line with your spine, it may help to place a folded towel between your arm and head.) Place the baby on a blanket with his body parallel to yours and his face near your head. Bend your knees so your thighs form a 45-degree angle with your hips. Planting your left hand on the floor in front of you for support, exhale as you lift your left leg to hip height. Inhale as you return the leg to the starting position. Do 8 to 12 reps. Turn onto your left side and repeat with your right leg. Work your way up to three sets.

Things to bear in mind: Keep your abdominals contracted through the move, don't roll your hips forward or backward, and keep your leg in the same plane as you lift—don't allow the knee to point up or down.

SIDE-LYING INNER THIGH LIFT

Muscles it targets: Inner thigh muscles (aka adductors).

Why do it: To firm up your inner thighs, which may be jiggly thanks to your ongoing weight loss.

How to do it correctly: Lie on your right side with your head resting comfortably on your right arm. (To keep your neck in line with your spine, it may help to place a folded towel between your arm and head.) Place the baby on a blanket with her body parallel to yours and her face near your head. Extend your right leg straight down. Bend your left knee and rest it in front of you on a pillow for support. Planting your left hand on the floor in front of you for support, exhale as you lift your left leg up as high as you can toward the ceiling without rolling your hips forward or backward. Inhale as you lower the leg to the starting position. Do 8 to 12 reps. Turn onto your left side and repeat with your right leg. Work your way up to three sets.

Things to bear in mind: Keep the foot of your lifted leg flexed and your toes facing forward, not up or down. Keep your pelvis in a neutral position and your spine straight.

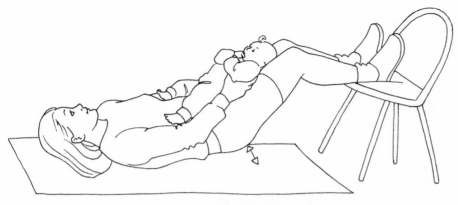

Butt Bridge

BUTT BRIDGE

Muscles it targets: Glutes and hamstrings.

Why do it: To tighten and firm your backside.

How to do it correctly: Lie on your back on the floor with your heels on the edge of a chair that's backed up to a wall for support. Rest your baby's butt against your pelvis and his head and back against your thighs. Hold on to him throughout the move. Holding in your abdominals, lift your rear end off the floor several inches. Feel the contraction in your butt and hamstrings. Lower your body to the starting position. Do 8 to 12 reps. Work your way up to three sets.

Things to bear in mind: To get the most out of this move, focus on the feeling of contraction in your butt and hamstrings. The movement is small; don't allow your back to leave the floor.

REVERSE AB CURL

Muscles it targets: Abdominals.

Why do it: To continue to strengthen your abs.

How to do it correctly: Lie on your back on the floor with the baby beside you in a bouncy seat or on a blanket. Place your hands, palms down, alongside your thighs. Bend your hips and knees to 90 degrees so your calves are parallel to the floor. Exhale as you slowly contract your abs, rolling your hips up off the floor 2 to 4 inches. Hold for 3 seconds. Inhale as you lower your butt slowly to the starting position. Do 8 to 12 reps. Work your way up to three sets.

Things to bear in mind: Don't move too quickly. To get the most out of this move, it needs to be done in a controlled manner. Don't cheat by pushing off with your arms, and don't lift your back off the mat. Keep your upper body and arms relaxed throughout the move.

How to Cope with Wrist Pain

Who knew that carrying around an 8-pound baby could be so hard on your body? Your back aches, your neck is sore—even your wrists feel tweaked.

Surprised? Don't be. That wrist and forearm pain is actually a form of carpal tunnel syndrome, which occurs commonly in the postpartum period as a result of holding the full weight of your infant in your arms while your wrist is bent. From now on, try to make sure your wrists are straight when you cradle your baby. Use a splint if you have to. If the problem continues, try the following strengthening moves:

• Sitting at a narrow table, hold a 2- or 3-pound weight in your hand. Lay your arm on the table with your palm up. Allow your wrist and hand to extend beyond the edge of the table. Then, slowly curl your hand toward the ceiling, and lower. Do 8 to 12 times, then repeat on the other side.

• Flip your arm over so your palm is facing down. Allow your wrist and hand to hang over the edge of the table. Then slowly flex your wrist so your knuckles point back toward your body, and lower. Do 8 to 12 times, then repeat on the other side.

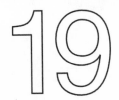

Enhancing Flexibility

Strengthening your muscles will do a lot for your physique in the coming months, but you'll still be left with a legacy of aches and pains unless you also stretch. While your ab muscles got longer and weaker during your pregnancy, your lower back muscles became shorter and tighter. Without some help, they'll stay that way. Other muscles that need tending in the coming months are those in your upper back and chest, your hamstrings, and your calves. And, if you're active (which we know you're going to be), you'll need to maintain a full-body stretching regimen to keep your muscles supple and resistant to strains.

The rules for stretching are much the same as those for strengthening. Ease into it slowly. You can start doing static, prone stretches from day one, but never stretch to the point of pain. Hold each stretch for 20 to 30 seconds at the point where you feel mild tension. Breathe normally throughout each move, and feel the tension flow out of your body when you release the stretch.

CALF, FOOT, AND ANKLE STRETCH (see chapter 15, page 149)

LOWER BACK STRETCH

Muscles it targets: Lower back and glutes.

Why do it: To start lengthening those tight lower back muscles and improve your posture.

How to do it correctly: Lying on your back, bend both knees with your feet flat on the floor about a foot apart. Pull your right knee toward your chest and loop a towel around your right foot. Keeping your foot flexed, bring your knee up toward your right shoulder, pulling gently with the towel. Hold for a count of three. Release. Do 5 reps. Repeat with the left leg.

When to do it: When you first wake up in the morning, before you go to sleep at night.

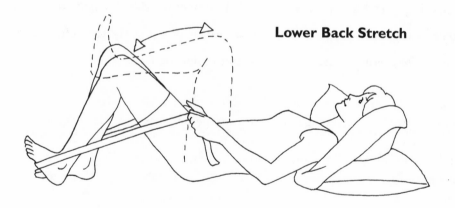

Lower Back Stretch

PRONE HAMSTRING STRETCH

Muscles it targets: Hamstrings.

Why do it: During pregnancy, your hamstrings became shorter and tighter. Now you need to lengthen them to give you a full range of motion in your pelvis and hips.

How to do it correctly: Lying on your back, bend both knees with your feet flat on the floor about a foot apart. Pull your right knee toward your chest and loop a towel around your right foot. Then straighten your right leg up in the air so the sole of your foot is pointing toward the ceiling. Keep your right knee soft. Use the towel to create a slight tension in the hamstring. Hold for 3 seconds. Lower the leg down to the floor. Do 5 reps. Repeat with the left leg.

When to do it: When you first wake up in the morning, before you go to sleep at night.

Weeks 2 to 4

Continue doing the stretches from the last two weeks, but add:

UPPER BODY STRETCH (see chapter 7, page 77)

CAT STRETCH

Muscles it targets: Erector spinae, lats, and traps.

Why do it: To release tension in your back and lengthen those tight muscles.

How to do it correctly: Kneel on all fours with your knees directly under your hips, your arms directly under your shoulders, and your spine straight. Exhale as you round your spine up toward the ceiling, allowing your tailbone and your head and neck to relax downward. Hold for a count of five. Return to the starting position. Do 5 reps.

When to do it: When the baby is lying on the floor playing, after a long day of carrying the baby around.

Continue doing the stretches from the past weeks and add the following.

TRICEPS STRETCH (see chapter 11, page 115)

BICEPS STRETCH

Muscles it targets: Biceps.

Why do it: To lengthen the muscles that are working hard to lift and carry the baby.

How to do it correctly: Extend your right arm out in front of you, palm facing up. With your left hand, pull the fingers of your right hand down toward the ground. Hold for a count of three. Do 5 sets. Repeat on the left arm.

When to do it: In the shower, before you pick up the baby in the morning, before you go to bed at night.

FULL CHEST STRETCH

Muscles it targets: Pecs and front of delts.

Why do it: To lengthen your chest muscles, which become shorter and tighter when you round your shoulders.

How to do it correctly: Holding on to both sides of a doorway with your hands at shoulder level, let your arms straighten as you lean your torso forward slightly.

When to do it: After you breast-feed or anytime you feel yourself slumping.

TRAPEZIUS STRETCH

Muscles it targets: Traps and lats.

Why do it: To relieve tension in the upper back, which can become tight and cramped from breast-feeding and carrying the baby.

How to do it correctly: Reach in front of you with both arms and clasp your hands gently together. Rounding your upper back slightly, press forward through your hands until you feel a slight stretch in your upper back. Hold for a count of three. Do 5 reps.

When to do it: After you breast-feed, before you pick up the baby in the morning, before you go to bed at night.

FULL BACK STRETCH (see chapter 15, page 147)

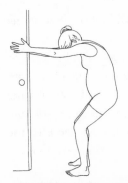

Full Back Stretch

QUADRICEPS STRETCH (see chapter 7, page 79)

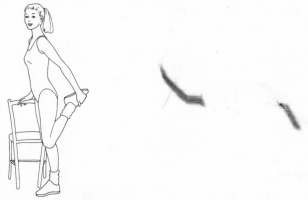

Quadriceps Stretch

CALF AND ACHILLES STRETCH (see chapter 7, page 81)

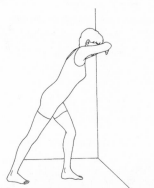

Calf and Achilles Stretch

TOE REACH

Muscles it targets: Erector spinae, hamstrings, and calves.

Why do it: To improve range of motion in your whole body and target the muscles that are most likely to be tight now.

How to do it correctly: Lean your back against a wall from buttocks to shoulders, but walk your feet out until they're about a foot and a half from the wall. With your feet parallel and hip-distance apart, bend forward at the hips, allowing your buttocks to slide up the wall. Keep your knees soft and allow your upper body to droop forward loosely, reaching as close to the floor as you can. Hold for 20 seconds. Roll up to the starting position one vertebra at a time.

When to do it: Before you pick up the baby in the morning, before you go to bed at night.

CHILD'S POSE (see chapter 15, page 148)

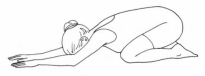

Child's Pose

ABDOMINAL STRETCH

Muscles it targets: Abdominals.

Why do it: Now that you're focusing so much on strengthening your abdominals, you need to be mindful of stretching them as well.

How to do it correctly: Lie on your back on the floor and extend your arms overhead. Reach your fingers and toes in opposite directions. Hold for 20 seconds.

When to do it: Before you get out of bed in the morning, after you do your ab work.

Afterword

Just as no one can prepare you for what it feels like to be pregnant, no one can prepare you for what it feels like to be a mother. A number of years ago there was a recruitment advertisement for the army that called it "The hardest job you'll ever love." That comes about as close to summing up motherhood as anything we've ever heard. It isn't easy. In fact, there may be times when you'd like to call your own mother or best friend or sister and scream, "Why didn't you tell me it would be this hard?" But after a good cry, you'll come to the same conclusion every other parent on the planet has ever come to: It's worth every sweaty, tearful, sleep-deprived minute of it. And guess what? It's easier if you continue to exercise.

Being physically fit gives you the stamina to chase down a toddler, teach a preschooler to ride a bike, coach soccer, or lead family hikes—to keep up with your kids as they grow into human beings you can enjoy in lots of different active environments. As importantly, regular exercise will continue to smooth out the rough edges, giving you the emotional agility to handle middle-of-the-night ear infections, produce-aisle tantrums, skinned knees, and bad report cards with more aplomb.

Ultimately, though, exercise isn't something you do to be a better parent, like taking a CPR class or being a Scout troop leader. In fact, there will be times when it's downright unpopular for Mommy to go for a run or to the gym, and there will be days (maybe lots of them) when you sacrifice your workout for the family's greater good. But keep this in mind: Parenthood is so demanding, it could easily swallow every nanosecond of your day if you don't lay down some ground rules and draw some clear boundaries. We suggest you carve out a niche for exercise in your life not for your kids, but for yourself.

The scientific research in favor of regular exercise couldn't be more convincing. In the last decade, doctors have found that weight-bearing exercise is one of the surest ways to stave off osteoporosis. Researchers also know vigorous cardiovascular exercise at least twice a week reduces the risk of heart disease. Stretching can help you maintain flexibility and avoid common aches and pains that come with the muscle rigidity of inactivity. Moreover, regular workouts can help you sustain muscle mass, keep your weight in check, improve your attitude, and increase your vitality. In short, exercise helps you age more healthfully, more attractively, more gracefully. And we can't think of a better way to go.

So, now that you've developed these good, pregnancy-inspired habits, why not extend them to the rest of your life? Use this book as a resource for at-home exercises (the moves we included are great for nonpregnant women as well), and don't forget to pull it out the minute you suspect you might be pregnant again. There's no reason to go through pregnancy—or life, for that matter—without feeling strong, healthy, and ready for anything.

Acknowledgments

I'm grateful to the editors of *Fitness* magazine for giving me the opportunity to write this book; Julie Merberg, my editor at Roundtable Press, who shepherded the project through the labyrinthine publishing system from beginning to end; and the fine folks at Clarkson Potter—John Son, Katie Workman, Camille Smith, Lauren Monchik, Maureen Clark, Robin Slutzky, and Lauren Shakely.

Huge hugs and snuggles to my two little guys, Will and Griffin, who taught me what pregnancy feels like from the inside out, and who remind me every day that running through sprinklers is as important as writing books. Thanks to my parents, who gave me Pulitzer-caliber praise for every terrible essay, poem, and book report I ever wrote, and to my mother-in-law, Dorothy Wright, for bragging about me in grocery store checkout lines.

My deepest appreciation goes to Gordon Wright, who is an exemplary father and an extraordinary husband: Who knew we'd ever get enough sleep to do productive work again? Thanks for being my mate, soul, and otherwise.

Ginny Graves

Recommended Reading

PREGNANCY EXERCISE BOOKS

Essential Exercises for the Childbearing Year, by Elizabeth Noble, New Life Images

Maternal Fitness, by Julie Tupler, Fireside Books

GENERAL EXERCISE BOOKS

The Complete Book of Fitness, by the editors of *Fitness* Magazine, Three Rivers Press

The Complete Book of Swimming, by Dr. Phillip Whitten, Random House

Fitness for Dummies, by Suzanne Schlosberg and Liz Neporent, IDG Books Worldwide, Inc.

Stretching, by Bob Anderson, Shelter Publications, Inc.

A Woman's Book of Strength, by Karen Andes, Perigee Books

Index